Tim Coltart, MA (Cantab), PhD ‾‾‾‾‾‾ (Lu), FRCOG, is the medical adviser to this book. He is a Consultant Obstetrician and Gynaecologist at Guy's Hospital and Queen Charlotte's & Chelsea Hospital, London. He has written extensively for medical textbooks and journals.

Felicity Smart, the author of this book, has edited many popular health publications. She is now a medical writer and this is her first book.

THE WOMAN'S
GUIDE
TO SURGERY

Felicity Smart
Medical Adviser, Tim Coltart

Thorsons
An Imprint of HarperCollinsPublishers

Thorsons
An Imprint of HarperCollins*Publishers*
77–85 Fulham Palace Road,
Hammersmith, London W6 8JB

Published by Thorsons 1992
10 9 8 7 6 5 4 3 2 1

© Felicity Smart 1992
Illustrations produced by the Department of
Audio Visual Services at Guy's Hospital, London

Felicity Smart asserts the moral right
to be identified as the author of this work

A catalogue record for this book
is available from the British Library

ISBN 0 7225 2577 X

Printed in Great Britain by
Billing & Sons Ltd, Worcester

Contents

Foreword

Surgical procedures for treating women's problems have under-
gone a revolution over the last ten years, offering greater choice
and effectiveness. When a woman visits her doctor or a specialist and is recommended to have an operation or investigation,
it will greatly help communication if she has an understanding
of her problem and its possible treatment. A thorough and
complete explanation cannot always be given at every consultation, and often it is not easy to 'take in' everything anyway
when you may be feeling tense and anxious. This is why *The
Woman's Guide to Surgery* is such a valuable source of information
and reassurance.

I am surprised that a book like this has not appeared before.
It can be read in your own time, for instance prior to a consultation, investigation or operation, to clarify any matters you
may want to discuss. It will also be helpful to have with you in
hospital and during recovery. Easy to read, this is a much-needed book. I can thoroughly recommend it.

Professor Stuart Campbell
Head of Obstetrics and Gynaecology
King's College Hospital, London

Acknowledgements

Our thanks are due to the following for their contributions to the writing of this book:

Mr Ian S. Fentiman, Consultant Surgeon, Clinical Oncology Unit, Guy's Hospital, London.

Mr M. A. Chaudary, Consultant Surgeon, Clinical Oncology Unit, Guy's Hospital, London.

Mr Hisham Hamed, Research Fellow, Clinical Oncology Unit, Guy's Hospital, London.

John Gold, Complementary Therapist and Counsellor.

Diana Moran, for permission to quote from her book *A More Difficult Exercise* (Bloomsbury, 1989).

Tim Coltart's personal thanks go to his secretary Julie Eagles; to David Bragg, Director of Audio Visual Services at Guy's Hospital, London; to Susanna Nasskau, the illustrator; and especially to his wife Eileen Coltart.

Felicity Smart's personal thanks go to Joy Langridge and Julie Eagles for their advice and kindness; to Sue Ferguson Linnell, Clare Ford, Sue Fleming and Judy Ridgway for their encouragement; to Jane Graham-Maw, Senior Editor at Thorsons, for her patience and help; to Barbara Vesey for her editorial expertise; to Susanna Nasskau for her excellent illustrations; to Nicola Williams for her perfect word-processing; to Marjorie Lampard for her brave example; and last, but far from least, to my dear husband Tim Smart, for his unfailing support.

Introduction

Most women will be recommended to have an operation or investigation at some time in their lives. This can come as a frightening shock when it happens to you—even if you were aware that your condition might one day need surgery. The fear can be made worse by the unknown. 'What's gone wrong?', 'What are they going to do to me?' and 'Will it hurt?' are the kind of alarming questions that can immediately well up. If it's a major operation, there's the additional anxiety about recovery and how much it will disrupt your life and the lives of those close to you. But the evidence is that the more you know about your problem, and what needs to be done about it, the better you will be able to deal with the whole experience of surgery.

Fear and anxiety make you tense; information and reassurance help you to relax. If you are calm, surgery of all types—whether major or minor—will not be such an ordeal, and you may actually recover faster from a major procedure.

The Woman's Guide to Surgery is here to help you feel as positive as possible. As the female author writing this introduction, I appreciated the need for this book when I had a major operation myself. I found there was no book to which I could refer that brought together the whole subject of surgery for women. I would have understood my problem, and its treatment, much more quickly if a book like this had existed. It would have enabled me to sort out the questions I needed to ask. I found that friends who'd had surgery felt as I did.

Being a general medical editor and writer, I decided to tackle this complex and specialized subject, and make it accessible in a straightforward way to other women. Tim Coltart, Consultant Obstetrician and Gynaecologist, has done much to help and advise me in writing the book and preparing the illustrations.

My own gynaecologist, Professor Stuart Campbell, completely understood the need to discuss my health problem fully so that the best decision on treatment could be made. He feels that this book will enable women and their doctors to communicate better.

The question-and-answer format is along the lines of a conversation you might want to have with your doctor or the specialist who treats you. It includes answers to the questions women most often ask—or may wish to ask but are hesitant to do so. We hope to reassure you and give you the confidence—if you need it—to put your own questions. You do have a right to information and choice regarding all aspects of your treatment. *The Woman's Guide to Surgery* will help you to exercise that choice.

A book such as this cannot, however, provide precise definitions. Surgical techniques can vary depending on the surgeon's opinion and the hospital's equipment. Treatments are also improved and new ones developed continually. This book therefore should be seen as a guide to the main techniques likely to be used. It covers a comprehensive range of 'invasive' procedures.

Beginning with the tests used in diagnosis, we explain minor surgical procedures and major operations. We take you through your hospital stay, giving advice on preparing for surgery and on recovery afterwards, if you need to convalesce. There is also extensive information on the disorders that can necessitate surgery. We also show how alternative therapies can benefit you: their value as a 'complement' to orthodox treatments is now increasingly recognized, especially in helping patients feel calm and relaxed. Being calm, confident and well-informed puts you more in control. We hope that *The Woman's Guide to Surgery* will give you the information you need to gain the greatest possible benefit from the medical advice you are given.

Index of
Starred* Items

To avoid repetition, key medical terms are starred* throughout the book. This quick-reference guide tells you where to find an explanation of each term.

1

DIAGNOSING WOMEN'S PROBLEMS

You're going for a check-up with your own doctor or at a clinic. Maybe you're simply having the routine tests that all women need. If so, you're very sensible; these tests are vital in preventing and diagnosing women's problems. Maybe you're going because you have worrying symptoms or are having difficulty becoming pregnant. If there is a problem — and don't just assume there must be — early diagnosis can make any treatment more effective.

Whatever your reasons for having a check-up, you're likely to be feeling apprehensive. This is quite usual, whether it's your first visit or you've been before. To help and reassure you, we shall describe what happens during a routine gynaecological or 'well woman' check-up, and why. We advise on how best to cope with any anxieties and embarrassment, and we explain the procedures most often used in diagnosis, some of which involve minor surgery. If you are well-informed, you will feel more confident and better able to ask questions and talk over any worries.

I feel perfectly well, so why is it sensible for me to have routine tests?

Because certain potentially serious disorders have few or no early symptoms but can be detected by tests. This doesn't mean you should worry about being ill if you feel perfectly well: most women are as healthy as they feel. But it is essential that the small minority who may be at risk are diagnosed early. This is why every woman has a responsibility to herself to have routine check-ups at the intervals recommended by her doctor. It is at this stage that you can do most to help and protect yourself.

If I have something seriously wrong with me, I'd rather not know.

The fear of finding out that 'something is wrong' is very common. For practically all women the greatest fear is, of course, of having cancer. We do stress that this fear is most often groundless – and in the unlikely event of there being anything seriously wrong, early diagnosis and treatment are certainly the best ways of dealing with it. Early diagnosis is also essential for certain infections of the reproductive tract, some of which can be sexually transmitted. If left untreated they can lead to major problems which may need surgery. The possibility of having a sexually transmitted infection often arouses considerable fear, embarrassment and even shame, but no woman should ever let such feelings prevent her from having a check-up. There is more about such infections on page 53. Failure to have routine checks and ignoring any symptoms will not make anything just 'go away'.

Are there any preparations I need to make before having a routine check-up?

Make sure that you will not be having a period at the time of your appointment, and don't use any contraceptive creams or gels the night before (if you have sex the night before and you are not on the pill your partner can use a condom). You may be asked to provide a urine sample – it's worth finding out about this in advance so you'll be in the right state to give one, if necessary; perhaps you can even bring one along with you. Wear clothes which you can get in and out of easily; you will need to undress above the waist for your breasts to be examined and below the waist for a pelvic examination, but you do not usually have to remove all your clothes at once.

What happens during a routine check-up?

First you will be asked questions about your health and medical history, if the doctor does not already have this information. Questions may also be asked about the health of close relatives, as this can sometimes be relevant to you.

This is followed by physical checks. The way in which a check-up is carried out can vary, depending on the opinion and approach of each individual doctor. Here is a general guide to what usually happens.

- You may be weighed and have your blood-pressure taken. A urine sample may be needed for testing, as already mentioned.
- The next stage is usually a breast examination. The appearance of your breasts is checked. This may be done while you are seated, although some doctors carry out the whole examination with the patient lying back on an examination couch, which is like a bed. Your breasts are gently pressed by hand (this is called palpation), and the doctor also feels both armpits carefully. This is to check for the presence of any lumps in the breasts or armpits. You will be shown how to do this for yourself, if you don't already know (see pages 223–4). You may be referred for mammography, which is a routine test (there is more about this later).
- This is followed by a pelvic examination. For this, you usually lie on your back with your knees bent and your feet comfortably apart – they may be supported by stir-rups – or you can lie on your side with your legs drawn up, if this more comfortable for you. Your bladder should be empty; a full bladder will impede the examination and be uncomfortable for you.

  The doctor starts by gently pressing your abdomen by hand (palpation) to feel for anything unusual. Then, wearing surgical gloves, s/he examines the vulva (the outer vaginal area) gently to check that there are no external problems.

This may be followed by a vaginal examination. The doctor inserts a speculum gently into your vagina, as illustrated below. This instrument is made of metal or plastic and looks like a duck's beak. It will be lubricated so it slips in easily, and a considerate doctor will ensure that it is not stone cold. It is hinged so that it can be opened and closed; it is closed when inserted and is then opened so that the vaginal walls and the cervix (the neck of the womb), which protrudes into the top of the vagina, can be seen clearly.

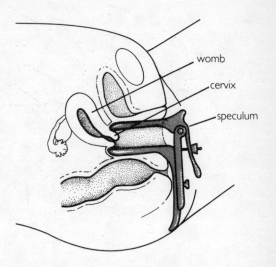

A speculum in place enables the vaginal walls and cervix to be seen.

The doctor will carry out a routine cervical smear test*. A wooden spatula or a special brush is used to remove some cells from the cervix — this only takes a few seconds. These cells will be sent for analysis to detect whether or not there are any abnormal changes to the cervix. The results most often show that everything is normal.

If there are any signs of infection, swabs will be taken: cotton swabs are wiped gently over the vaginal walls and cervix to pick up secretions. The swabs are then sent for analysis. A vaginal examination lasts only a few minutes; the speculum is then removed.

- A bi-manual (two-handed) pelvic examination is combined
  with the vaginal examination: the doctor slips one or two
  fingers, which have been lubricated, into the vagina and
  again presses the abdomen gently with the other hand. The
  pelvic organs – the womb, ovaries and Fallopian tubes –
  can thus be felt, and the doctor can tell whether everything
  is normal. It is helpful if you are not overweight because it
  is then easier for the doctor to feel the pelvic organs.

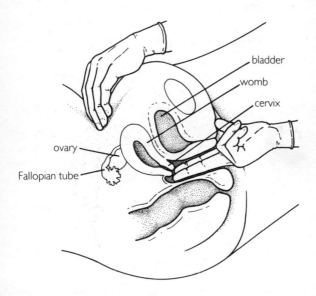

A routine bi-manual (two-handed) pelvic examination.

*You say that a bi-manual pelvic examination is combined with the vaginal
examination. Which is usually carried out first?*

Whether the bi-manual or the vaginal examination is carried out
first depends on the doctor. S/he may start by looking inside
the vagina using the speculum; if swab tests are then needed
they won't pick up the lubricant which s/he used when doing a
bi-manual. But a doctor will sometimes start with the bi-manual
because it may be easier for the woman – particularly if she is a
new patient – than having a speculum inserted straight away. It

is also a way of reassuring her by gentle touch before an instrument is used.

Will any of this be painful?

No, it shouldn't hurt at all, but if you are tense an internal examination may be uncomfortable because your vaginal muscles will grip the speculum. Try to relax. A cervical smear test may cause a little discomfort, but some women hardly feel it at all. Sometimes the ovaries can be sensitive when felt during a bi-manual, so too can the womb when the cervix is moved; this is normal, but if you feel any pain during an examination, tell the doctor immediately.

I feel embarrassed and nervous about having a pelvic examination and being asked intimate personal questions. How can I cope with these feelings?

Such feelings generally arise because the most private and sexual areas of the body are on view to the doctor, who may be a stranger — and a man, since the majority of doctors and specialists are men, although an increasing number now are women. If you are attending a clinic which has several doctors, you could ask to see a woman doctor if you prefer, but you would need to ask in advance and it might not be possible. Also, some women can feel just as embarrassed with a woman doctor.

How can you cope with these feelings? First of all, you can reduce the 'embarrassment factor' by telling yourself that to a doctor a woman's most private anatomy is a familiar sight and that you will not be judged in a personal way. Similarly, all the answers you give to the doctor's questions will be treated in the strictest confidence and, again, no personal judgements will be passed on you. Doctors are used to hearing very personal details, and it is important for your own sake that you give full and honest answers. You can take a partner, relation or friend with you, but sometimes it is actually easier to be frank and talk over any anxieties when you are alone with the doctor.

You will not be expected to undress in front of the doctor

before being examined. S/he will either leave the room, or you can go behind a screen. In a clinic you may be asked to undress before seeing the doctor and will be given a dressing gown to put on. As mentioned earlier, it's not usually necessary to remove all your clothes at once.

While you are waiting to see the doctor you can help reduce any anxiety by closing your eyes and relaxing, breathing in deeply and breathing out slowly. Alternatively, talking to other patients who are waiting can be reassuring.

Should I tell the doctor about my feelings?

Yes. Most doctors will do their best to put you at ease. Doctors are professionals, and throughout an examination will concentrate on gaining thorough and accurate information on the state of your health. But there is an increasing awareness among doctors that their job is more than just technical. Having the doctor explain the examination as it progresses is often very helpful and reassuring, as you will know what to expect next. If necessary, ask him or her to do this.

To further reassure a patient, the doctor may have a female nurse present during the examination, although this is not always the case. You can request that a nurse be present, if you wish.

Are there any ways I can reassure myself?

Some women are reassured by being able to see as much of an examination as possible, although others prefer not to. A sheet or blanket is placed over you which hides the lower half of your body during the examination, but you can remove it if you want to see more of what is going on.

A way of familiarizing yourself with your own body, which may reduce any feelings of embarrassment, is to carry out an internal self-examination from time to time. How you do this is explained at the end of the chapter, but keep in mind that this is no substitute for a proper medical check.

What should I do if I can't get on with the doctor who examines me?

Some of us do encounter doctors or specialists whom we find it difficult to get on with. This doesn't necessarily mean they are any less good medically, but if you find it impossible to relax and communicate with a particular doctor, you should change to another. If you are attending a clinic, ask to see someone else.

Could you describe the sort of symptoms I should have checked? I don't like to bother my doctor unnecessarily.

If you have a good doctor, s/he will not make you feel you are being a bother, so if you have worrying symptoms, make an appointment. It won't take long for the doctor to tell you whether you are worrying unnecessarily. Symptoms which must be checked are as follows:

- periods which are heavy, painful or irregular
- any bleeding between periods or after the menopause
- persistent pelvic pain, feelings of heaviness and distention
- pain or bleeding during or after sex
- any unusual vaginal discharge which is heavy, discoloured, blood-stained, irritating or unpleasant smelling
- inflammations and irritations of the vagina and vulva
- swelling in the groin, i.e. a lump or lumps
- burning or pain on urination; increased frequency of urination
- any changes in the appearance of the breasts, such as puckered skin
- persistent pain in the breasts
- discharge from the nipples, yellowish or blood-stained
- inverted or cracked nipples, the nipple 'pulling' to one side
- a rash on the breast or nipple
- finding a lump in the breast
- swelling under the arm (a lump or lumps)

Yet again, we do stress that these symptoms do not necessarily indicate anything sinister, but they certainly must not be 'put up with' or ignored.

What will happen if I go to the doctor with any of these symptoms?

If the doctor thinks it necessary, you will be referred to a specialist for further investigation. Problems 'below the waist' are the concern of either a gynaecologist (and gynaecologists are also surgeons) or a specialist in genito-urinary medicine. In Britain, breast problems are the concern of a general surgeon specializing in breast disease; elsewhere they may also be treated by a gynaecologist. If you are referred to a specialist, this doesn't mean that surgery is inevitable. The specialist will examine you and discuss your symptoms with you. You may then be recommended to have certain diagnostic procedures.

Could you explain exactly what 'certain diagnostic procedures' means?

This depends on your symptoms, but below we explain the procedures most often used to diagnose the causes of women's problems.

D & C (dilation and curettage)

A D & C is the most common minor surgical procedure needed by women; the majority need it at some time in their lives. It is sometimes called 'diagnostic curettage'.

WHY IT IS NEEDED
The purpose of a D & C is to biopsy (take samples) of the endometrium (lining of the womb) for examination under a microscope; it is a form of endometrial biopsy. A D & C is carried out for a variety of reasons: to find the causes of heavy, painful or irregular periods, bleeding between periods, bleeding during or after sex, and after the menopause.

One of its uses is to investigate possible cancerous changes to the cervix or womb, but if you have any of the worrying symptoms just mentioned, don't assume you must have cancer. The causes can include a hormone imbalance*, which may respond to hormone treatment, or benign growths such as polyps* or fibroids*, which can also be treated.

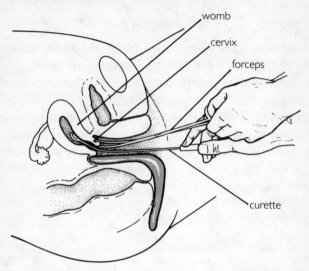

In a D & C (dilation and curettage), the cervix is widened (dilated) and samples of womb lining removed by curette for examination.

A D & C has other uses as well. It can be used not only to investigate polyps, but to remove them. Any remnants of a miscarriage* or of the placenta* after childbirth can be cleared by D & C. It can be part of infertility* investigations: examining the womb lining can help determine why a woman has difficulty in conceiving.

HOW IT IS CARRIED OUT

At most a D & C requires only an overnight stay in hospital, but it can often be carried out on a day-patient basis (see the next chapter). It is usually done under general anaesthetic, but a local anaesthetic may be used; if so this will be injected into the cervix. The vagina is held open with a speculum so the cervix can be seen. The cervix is the entrance to the womb, and it needs to be dilated (widened) so the womb lining can be removed. The cervix is steadied so that metal rods (dilators) can be inserted into the cervix to dilate it. A spoon-shaped instrument called a curette is then passed into the womb so the lining can be gently scraped. The whole procedure takes only 10 to 15 minutes.

AFTER-EFFECTS
You may have some bleeding and mild period-like cramps for a day or two following a D & C. Use sanitary towels (not tampons, because these increase the risk of infection). Don't have sex until any bleeding stops. Periods may be irregular for a couple of months while the womb lining returns to its normal functioning (see page 47), but contraception is needed right away. There are no long-term effects, and most women resume their normal lives the day after a D & C.

Suction curettage

Suction curettage can be another way of performing an endometrial biopsy (removing samples of womb lining for examination).

WHY IT IS NEEDED
Like a D & C, suction curettage is used in diagnosis to find the causes of abnormal bleeding. The gynaecologist may choose to carry out this procedure rather than a D & C for several reasons. A biopsy by suction curettage can be done without any anaesthetic, unlike a D & C, and so would be suitable for a woman who is not fit enough for an anaesthetic. If a woman has had children, the cervix is naturally less tight, and so it is simple to perform. The surgeon's decision may also depend on the patient's reaction; a woman who is nervous is more likely to prefer a D & C under general anaesthetic to having an endometrial biopsy without anaesthetic.

HOW IT IS CARRIED OUT
Suction curettage is performed in the out-patient clinic of a hospital. A very fine metal or plastic tube is inserted into the womb via the cervix, which does not need to be dilated beforehand. Low-pressure vacuum suction is applied to the

tube, allowing samples of womb lining to be withdrawn. This may be a little uncomfortable at the time, but takes only a few minutes.

AFTER-EFFECTS
After-effects are similar to but milder than those of a D & C.

Hysteroscopy

Hysteroscopy is quite a new procedure. It allows the gynaecologist a direct look inside the womb. It is carried out using a hysteroscope, a small instrument about as thick as a pencil with a light and a telescopic lens at one end. There can be several channels in it; one for looking down, another through which fluid or gas can be introduced into the womb (this is done to separate the walls of the womb to give a better view inside) – there may also be a channel through which fine instruments can be passed into the womb for minor surgery.

WHY IT IS NEEDED
Hysteroscopy has a number of uses. It may be carried out on its own as an investigative procedure, or be used together with minor surgical procedures. For instance, it enables the surgeon to locate polyps* in the womb before doing a D & C to remove them; the surgeon can then check again afterwards to see whether the D & C has been successful. Forceps can be passed down a channel in the hysteroscope to biopsy samples of womb lining for examination.

Hysteroscopy is also used in endometrial ablation* or resection*. These minor surgical procedures were developed recently. They can permanently remove the womb lining; this means that it does not grow again, as it does after a biopsy. The woman ceases to have periods, or they are only very light. These procedures are therefore used to resolve heavy, painful periods, if hormone treatment has not worked (see Chapter 3, on Resolving Period Problems). A hysteroscope enables the surgeon to perform either procedure accurately.

HOW IT IS CARRIED OUT

If hysteroscopy is carried out on its own, it can be done under sedation and a local anaesthetic — although of course a general anaesthetic is needed if it is carried out with other procedures which require one. The cervix needs to be dilated only slightly so the hysteroscope can be inserted into the womb.

AFTER-EFFECTS

There are no after-effects from hysteroscopy alone.

Ultrasound

Ultrasound is a diagnostic technique carried out externally, which means that no surgery is involved and no anaesthetic needed. It's a way of viewing (or scanning) pelvic organs, and is carried out at a hospital or clinic on an out-patient basis (see illustration).

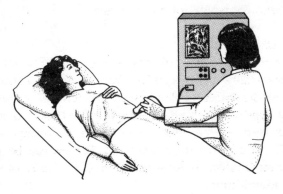

Ultrasound is a completely painless external procedure, enabling the pelvic organs to be viewed on a video monitor.

WHY IT IS NEEDED

Ultrasound shows up such problems as fibroids*, ovarian tumours* and displacement of pelvic organs. Another use is in infertility testing* to check whether ovulation* is taking place (i.e. that the woman's ovaries are producing eggs). During pregnancy it is used to monitor the development of the fetus. It can also be used as a guide when other diagnostic procedures are performed, particularly during pregnancy (see page 71–5). It can also show whether breast lumps are solid or fluid-filled, and it may be used to detect breast cancer in women under 50.

HOW IT IS CARRIED OUT

To have an abdominal ultrasound scan, you need to remove the clothes from your lower abdomen. It may not be necessary to undress, just to push your clothes down over your hips, although this depends on the method used. Oil or jelly is then applied to your abdomen to ensure that the instrument the doctor uses, called a transducer, has maximum contact with your skin. The doctor moves the transducer slowly back and forth over your abdomen.

What is happening is that high-frequency sound waves (which cannot be heard) are reflected off pelvic organs and translated into images on a video monitor. It's fascinating to watch – the doctor will explain which organs are on view – and there is no discomfort. It only takes 15 minutes, or even less.

You may need to have a full bladder, because this separates the pelvic organs, making them easier to see. If you are not already in this state, you will be given a jug of water and a glass, and be asked to drink as much as possible. Increasingly, however, special ultrasound probes are being used which fit comfortably into the vagina and give better pictures; you won't need a full bladder for this method, but you will need to undress fully below the waist.

For a breast scan, oil or jelly is applied to the breast and the transducer used to pick up images, as already described.

The oil/jelly used in ultrasound is simply wiped off afterwards, and does not stain clothes.

AFTER-EFFECTS

Ultrasound is considered to be completely safe, and there are no known after-effects.

Laparoscopy

Laparoscopy is a minor surgical procedure which enables the pelvic organs to be seen directly. A laparoscope is a telescopic instrument no wider than an average ball-point pen, which has a light at one end.

WHY IT IS NEEDED

Laparoscopy is used to investigate the causes of pelvic pain when these are not made obvious by a pelvic examination. Pain can be caused by inflammation resulting from infection. If the inflammation becomes long standing it is known as chronic pelvic inflammatory disease (PID)*. Pain may also be due to endometriosis*, the disorder where patches of womb lining are present outside the womb in the pelvis and cause painful inflammation, especially during periods. Or pain may have other causes, such as an ectopic pregnancy*, where the fetus has lodged outside the womb, usually in the Fallopian tube.

Laparoscopy also has other purposes. Ovarian tumours* can be investigated and biopsied. It can be used to inspect the Fallopian tubes when the causes of infertility* are being diag-nosed (see illustration). Eggs can be removed from the ovaries by laparoscopy so they can be fertilized outside the womb and then implanted back into the womb. This is known as the 'test tube baby' technique or, more accurately, as in vitro fertilization (IVF)*. It can overcome infertility caused by blocked Fallopian tubes or as a result of the tubes having been removed. Conversely, laparoscopy is also used in sterilization*. New methods using the laparoscope are continually being developed to replace formal operations.

HOW IT IS CARRIED OUT

Laparoscopy is usually performed under general anaesthetic (although a local can be used) in hospital and you will probably need to be in overnight. The procedure requires two small inci-sions in the abdomen, one almost in the navel and the other near the pubic hairline. Both are no more than 1 cm (½ in) long and leave only very small scars. First, harmless carbon dioxide gas is pumped into the abdomen via a fine needle. This inflates the abdomen and separates the intestines from the pelvic organs, making them easier to see. The laparoscope is then inserted via the incision in the navel. Instruments designed to carry out minor surgery, IVF or sterilization can be inserted through the lower incision.

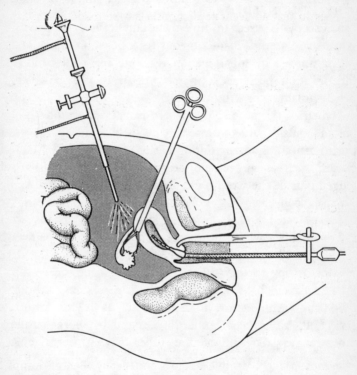

The pelvic organs being viewed by laparoscope inserted just below the navel into the abdomen, which is first inflated with harmless gas. Surgical instruments can then be inserted just above the pubic hairline. When testing for infertility, a dye may be introduced into the womb via a tube in the vagina (shown here) to see whether the Fallopian tubes are open.

AFTER-EFFECTS

The gas in the abdomen may cause you some discomfort, and you may feel some pain in the shoulders 'referred' there via nerves that connect with the diaphragm. This is called 'referred pain'. It will go away once the gas has been absorbed by the

body – usually within a couple of days. There are no other
after-effects.

Breast biopsy

Breast biopsy is also a minor surgical procedure. As with other
biopsies, its purpose is to remove a small sample of tissue for
analysis so that an accurate diagnosis can be made.

WHY IT IS NEEDED
A general surgeon will biopsy a breast lump to find out whether
or not it is cancerous, but if you are having this done, don't
panic. **The vast majority of breast lumps are benign.**

HOW IT IS CARRIED OUT
A breast biopsy is performed either by 'cutting needle' or 'needle aspiration'. These are both done under local anaesthetic at a
hospital out-patient clinic. In cutting needle biopsy, a special
hollow needle is inserted through the skin into the lump and a
tiny cylinder of tissue is 'cored out' and withdrawn with the
needle. In needle aspiration, the needle is attached to a syringe
and a few cells are sucked out under low pressure. Both these
procedures are called 'closed' operations because skin and tissue
are not cut and only a very small puncture mark is left on the
skin.

Sometimes a breast lump may be biopsied as an 'open' operation under general anaesthetic in hospital. The whole lump will
be removed and a sample tested immediately. Benign lumps do
not require any further surgery, but if a lump is found to be
cancerous the surgeon may want to proceed with the appropriate surgery right away while the woman is still under anaesthetic. This means that you would need to give your consent
to surgery beforehand, and that the surgeon will have discussed
the options with you. Out-patient 'closed' biopsies are now so
reliable, however, that it is often unnecessary to perform open
surgery, which means that the diagnosis can be fully considered
before the woman consents to surgery, rendering it less traumatic for her. See Chapter 16, on Breast Surgery.

X-ray

X-ray is a very well known method of diagnosis which has many uses. Virtually everyone will have had an X-ray of some part of the body at one time or another. It is a means of taking highly accurate pictures of the inside of the body using electromagnetic radiation. Great care is taken to control exposure to radiation, as it is harmful in large doses. An X-ray lasts only a fraction of a second, and you feel nothing at all.

X-ray is not only useful in diagnosis. Electromagnetic radiation also has the power to destroy cancer cells when they are bombarded with X-rays, and so is used in radiotherapy* to treat cancer.

USES OF X-RAY IN DIAGNOSING WOMEN'S PROBLEMS

- **Mammography** (as X-raying the breast is called) detects breast lumps and is valuable in showing up tumours which are too small to be felt, so they can be treated early. In Britain it is recommended for all women over 50 and for women over 40 with a family history of breast cancer*.
- **Hysterosalpingography** is a means of X-raying the inside of the womb and the Fallopian tubes when testing for the causes of infertility*.
- **CT scanning** produces cross-sectional images of the body in 'slices', so that a complete picture can be built up. This is particularly useful in detecting the spread of cancer. CT scanning involves undressing and putting on a surgical gown, then lying on a special table which passes into the scanner. The body is X-rayed from different angles and the images are co-ordinated by a computer. Again, you don't feel anything, although some people find it claustrophobic inside the scanner; closing your eyes and concentrating on relaxing your whole body will help.

If I have any of these diagnostic procedures, what will happen next?

This depends on the results, which you will receive either from your own doctor or direct from the clinic or hospital.

Often no further treatment is necessary, sometimes drugs may be prescribed, but in other instances surgery will be recommended.

Supposing I am recommended to have an operation, can I ask questions about it?

Yes, you certainly can ask questions about it, if you want to, and this book will help you to discuss the operation with your doctor or specialist. If you are in any doubt about having an operation, you can always ask your doctor to refer you to another specialist for a second opinion. You are not obliged to have any treatment at all, if you don't want it, although you must consider carefully the reasons why it is advisable – again, this book should help you do this.

The next chapter will inform and reassure you about preparing for surgery.

I've heard that it's possible to have symptoms, such as chronic pelvic pain, for which no cause can be found. What should a woman do if this happens?

Sometimes symptoms of chronic pelvic pain, and also vaginal irritation and discharge, can occur without a physical cause being found. Stress or emotional upset can produce such symptoms as a result of the mind influencing the body; these are known as psychosomatic symptoms. However, all the possible physical causes must be investigated fully before this diagnosis is made (certain painful disorders, such as endometriosis* and PID*, can be difficult to diagnose).

If no physical cause of a woman's symptoms is found, it would be worthwhile for her to have counselling. Her doctor can put her in touch with a counsellor (see also the Useful Addresses section at the end of this book). Counselling can help to uncover the underlying problem and resolve it.

Should I carry out the internal self-examination mentioned earlier?

For some women, being familiar with their own body is a way of overcoming ignorance and embarrassment about it. Some women also choose to carry out internal self-examination together with other women in a self-help group because it gives them further reassurance. This can help them to feel more confident about going for medical checks, but – as already said – it cannot be a substitute for regular check-ups. Not all women want to examine themselves, and it is entirely a matter of choice, so only do it if you think it will help you.

How is an internal self-examination done?

It's a simple procedure. All you need is a plastic speculum (obtainable from surgical suppliers), a hand mirror, a small flashlight and some lubricating jelly. Open and close the speculum a few times to see how it works. Then lubricate it and, sitting comfortably with your legs apart, insert it, holding the handle upwards. Open it until it clicks into position. You will then be able to see inside the vagina, using the flashlight and the mirror. Remove the speculum while it is still open; otherwise you may pinch yourself. Wash the speculum afterwards using an antiseptic soap.

If I examine myself, what should I look for?

Just note your internal appearance and the state of vaginal secretions at different times of the month. They will be thick and creamy before and after your fertile time (ovulation*) and thinner, stringier and wetter at ovulation (which allows sperm through so that fertilization can take place – that is, if you are not using contraception).

Your cervix is the round, pink protrusion at the top of your vagina; tensing your stomach muscles can make it more visible. If you are pregnant it will be bluish and its secretions heavier; taking the pill also produces a bluish colour because its effect is to imitate the signs of pregnancy. During breastfeeding there are less secretions, and so the cervix looks drier. After the menopause it is also drier and a much paler pink in colour.

Regular internal self-examination can help you to note any unusual changes, should these occur, so that you can report them to your doctor promptly. But you shouldn't carry out a self-examination anxiously expecting to find trouble. It is simply a routine health care measure which can be part of taking a positive attitude to your body.

2

PREPARING FOR SURGERY

You've been advised to have an operation or investigation in hospital under general anaesthetic. Even if you were expecting this, you're still likely to be feeling anxious. If you've had surgery before you will of course have a better idea of what to expect, but whether or not this is the case few women ever 'sail through' without worry. Waiting for surgery can almost be the worst part; this is when fears are often uppermost, and reassurance so vital.

Some women prefer to be told as little as possible, simply needing the assurance that 'everything will be all right'. For the increasing number of women who want to know how best to help themselves, however, we offer a step-by-step guide through the necessary preparations and advice on how to keep as relaxed and positive as possible.

I'm awaiting admission to hospital for an operation. How can I use the time constructively?

In two important ways. Firstly, by improving your morale (and, if possible, your general health), you will feel more capable of coping physically and emotionally with surgery. Secondly, by organizing the practical side of your life, so that you won't find yourself worrying about things going on at home or at work while you are in hospital.

I feel increasingly anxious and afraid. Is there anything I can do about this?

To start with, accept that it is normal to feel like this. Going into hospital for surgery is certainly a stressful experience for just about everyone, and most people also feel particularly scared the day before surgery. This is why improving your morale is so important. Stress undermines us physically and emotionally, so if you can find ways of reducing stress you will be less sensitive to any pain and be more likely to make a quick recovery.

Tell me how I can reduce stress and boost my morale.

Fear and anxiety are often caused by ignorance and uncertainty. When any fears and anxieties you have are dispelled, you will very likely feel a lot more positive. Doctors and nurses are aware of this, but they cannot always know what is worrying you. So don't hesitate to ask questions. There is evidence that the better informed most patients are, the better they are able to cope.

Doctors and nurses are sometimes criticized, however, for not being sufficiently good at communication. Equally, some patients are not particularly good at communicating their anxieties. This is where this book can be most helpful. Reading the chapter relevant to your particular condition and its treatment will give you essential information and help you to decide what questions you need to ask.

If you are having a major operation, such as a hysterectomy* (removal of the womb), you will of course need more advice and support than if you are having a minor procedure, such as a D & C (dilation and curettage)*. Counselling and support groups exist to help women who are facing major surgery, or recovering from it. Ask your doctor or hospital about these and see the Useful Addresses section.

When you say I should improve my general health, do you mean through diet and exercise?

Yes, but also by maintaining a balance between mind and body, so that you are calm and relaxed. Relaxation techniques, massage and Yoga can all be very helpful. Read Chapter 18 on

Alternative Therapies and Healthier Living for further advice. Do also ask your doctor, who may give advice specific to your needs. But there are two very important matters concerning physical health which must be included here, because they relate directly to surgery.

1. If you are overweight this can make abdominal operations technically more difficult to perform. If a patient is very overweight, the surgeon may even be influenced against attempting certain operations because of the risks involved. Being overweight means that healing takes longer after surgery and the risks of the wound becoming infected are greater. It is a fact that people who are not overweight heal better and recover faster. So if your doctor or surgeon advises you to lose weight, you would be very wise to use the time before surgery to lose some weight through careful dieting and exercise.

2. Smoking is not only damaging to health, it also carries particular risks following surgery. A smoker is at greater risk of developing chest complications and pneumonia after being under a general anaesthetic. This is because smokers produce more mucus in the bronchial tubes of their lungs. After an operation, patients are reluctant to cough (it hurts and can disrupt the stitches), so in a smoker the mucus won't be removed and therefore stagnates, leading to infection. If you smoke, it is therefore well worth trying to quit in preparation for surgery. People who manage to do this often find they have kicked the habit for good. You will not be allowed to smoke in hospital anyway, except in the day-room or outside the ward, unless of course you are in a private room.

I am going into hospital shortly. What preparations do I need to make?

The hospital's letter of admission will give you information, and you may also be sent a booklet, or there may be leaflets available, which can help you. Here are some general guidelines.

1. Remember that for most gynaecological operations (surgery on the reproductive tract: the womb, ovaries and vagina) you must not be having a period at the time of surgery, so check the dates when yours is due – unless, of course, you are past the menopause. Notify your doctor or the hospital if the proposed date is unsuitable.

2. Also notify your doctor or the hospital if you have a cold or any other ailment, as this might make surgery inadvisable.

3. If you are on the combined oestrogen/progestogen contraceptive pill, you will need to come off it at least a month before a major operation. This is because oestrogen encourages blood clots to form after surgery. It isn't necessary to stop taking it before a minor procedure. It is also safe to continue taking the progestogen-only minipill, whether you are having major or minor surgery.

4. If you are taking HRT* (hormone replacement therapy) to help with menopausal symptoms*, you may be advised to discontinue it before major surgery, although for the most part this will not be necessary.

5. For a minor surgical procedure you may be treated as a day-patient, which means you will not be staying in hospital overnight. You won't need to take any items in with you; just arrive at the right time and place. Do however arrange to have transport available, particularly to take you home afterwards. You may need a day to recover, so ensure that for two days any domestic matters will be taken care of, such as the shopping, looking after the children and cooking meals.

6. If you will be in hospital for longer than a day (you are likely to be in for about a week after a major operation), you will need to take nightwear, washing things, and other items such as paper tissues, talc and a cologne stick or spray – much the same as you would need in a hotel. You may also want to take in some books and magazines, and a radio (if it has an earpiece or headphones), although the hospital may provide this. You may find that the hospital has its own radio station. This has been

found to be very successful in raising patients' morale. Programmes may include putting patients in touch with each other via chat shows and playing their special music requests. You could also take in a cassette player with headphones so you can listen to your favourite tapes. If you have a very small portable TV you may be allowed to use it, if it comes with headphones.

Being in hospital is a good opportunity to do such things as sewing, knitting, crochet or embroidery, if you enjoy them; they will also help pass the time before and after the operation. If you are going to write letters or cards, take stationery, a pen and stamps. You will also be able to buy most of these things, if necessary, from the hospital shops or ward trolley when it comes round, so a little money will be useful. Have some change for making phone calls, although in a private room there will be a telephone by the bed and any calls will be charged to your account. Don't take in anything valuable, such as jewellery or a watch (though a plastic one will be all right).

Photos of loved ones by the bed – and even that old teddy bear – will cheer you up (you'd be surprised at how many patients have a cuddly mascot with them in hospital, so don't feel foolish about this!).

7. Again, make arrangements beforehand for transport to and from the hospital. Try to have someone with you – a partner, relative or friend – especially when you are going home. The hospital may be able to help with transport, if you have any difficulty.

8. We have already mentioned domestic matters. If you will be in hospital for more than a day or two, and may need to convalesce afterwards, it is vital to ensure that you are organized at home. Before going into hospital, make any arrangements necessary for the care of family members and pets. You may need a home help, but this will depend on how much a partner, relatives and friends can do. Hospitals have medical social workers who can help sort out any practical problems, particularly if you are

admitted at short notice. If you live alone, do lock your home securely, and have the keys with you in hospital.

9. If you have a job, make sure your employer is fully aware of your situation. Also ensure that you can claim any sickness benefits due to you.

10. Give some thought to the matter of visitors. You will not be feeling at all well straight after the operation and very probably won't want to see anyone then, except perhaps a partner or someone close to you; let other people know this in advance. You may tire easily for a while afterwards, so be prepared to tell visitors if you're not up to talking or to seeing them. If possible, arrange for one person to let the others know how you are. In a ward where other patients could be disturbed by noise, you may not be allowed more than two visitors at a time anyway. Voluntary workers and ministers of religion make regular visits to hospitals. They are sensitive to patients' feelings and will probably be aware of whether or not you want to talk to them, but – again – don't hesitate to make your wishes clear. On the positive side, visitors, 'get well' cards and flowers are all good for morale and can help in recovery, so don't 'shut people out' unless you feel you really have to.

Can you describe what will happen when I am admitted to hospital?

There is no set procedure which applies to every hospital, but this is what is likely to happen.

1. The letter of admission you receive will of course give you the date and time to arrive, and tell you where to go in the hospital. On arrival, admission forms need to be filled in and you will be given an identity bracelet with your name on it. Don't take this off until you have left hospital.

2. You may be asked to get ready for bed right away, because a doctor will come to examine you and this will be easier if you are already undressed.

3. The doctor who examines you will make routine checks, such as your blood-pressure, heart and lungs. A blood sample may also be taken. You will be asked questions about your medical history, and about any medicines you are taking or any allergies you may have. This is to ensure that the proposed treatment will be safe for you. You will be required to hand over any medicines you have with you; they will be given you as needed.

4. Discussing your operation with you is a very important part of the doctor's visit, even though you will have talked about it before with your own doctor and the specialist. This is done to make absolutely sure you understand the procedure and are in agreement with it. You may find it helpful to have this book with you. It would also be a good idea to write down any questions you may have; this will ensure that you can't forget what it was you meant to ask. Your surgeon (who may be your Consultant) and the anaesthetist may visit you too. Take these opportunities to ask questions as well.

5. You will then be asked to sign a form consenting to the operation. Again, be absolutely certain you understand this. Read it carefully and don't hurry. You have a right to ask for the consent form to be explained to you, and the hospital has a duty to do this. You are not obliged to consent to anything if you don't want to and you don't have to sign the form. Your treatment can always be discussed further with you and, if necessary, be reconsidered. You also have the right to leave hospital at any time if you want to.

6. You won't be given anything to eat or drink for at least four hours before surgery. This it to eliminate any possibility of your inhaling vomit if you are sick under the anaesthetic, although this rarely happens. If your operation is in the morning, you will be admitted to hospital the day before and can have an evening meal but no breakfast. For an operation in the afternoon or evening, you will be admitted in the morning or early afternoon and can have a light meal. If you are admitted as an

emergency case and have recently eaten, the hospital will try and wait four hours before operating to allow the stomach time to empty; if this is not possible, then each hospital has a safety routine to cope with such situations. Should you be unable to sign the consent form, then a partner, relative or other responsible person can do so.

7. In a teaching hospital, you may find that the Consultant visits you with a small group of medical students. They will discuss your case and may want to ask you questions and examine you. If you don't want to go along with this you can say so; you are under no obligation to agree to it. But if you feel you can co-operate, you may find it interesting and you will have helped to educate the next generation of doctors. You might also be asked to take part in a research project – again, this is entirely up to you.

I feel very nervous about going into hospital. Am I being cowardly?

No. Hospitals, particularly the larger ones, can seem impersonal and intimidating. Patients can feel vulnerable because hospital is a place where they may have to endure unpleasant things. But, as we have said, you are likely to feel more confident if you know what you are 'in for', in every sense. Remember too that you are still an individual with rights.

Once you're in your ward or room and have talked to the doctors and nurses you will probably begin to feel more secure. The time spent waiting for surgery will pass more easily if you read, listen to the radio or watch TV (there is usually a set in the day-room, and there will be one provided in a private room). If you find you can't concentrate enough for these, sewing, knitting, crochet or embroidery can be soothing, as already suggested. Or you may just want to meditate, think, or pray.

For many people, one of the most rewarding and reassuring aspects of being in hospital is getting to know the other patients. Everyone is 'in the same boat' as you, and this can create a great feeling of solidarity, which can more than compensate for any perceived loss of privacy or dignity. Patients can be very supportive of one another and are often helpful in practical ways. Lasting friendships are sometimes formed as a result of shared hospital experiences.

I am afraid I won't be able to sleep in hospital, particularly on the night before my operation.

You can of course have sleeping pills, but you could try the relaxation techniques described on page 265 to see if they work for you. In a ward there are likely to be disturbances during the night, necessary to the care of patients after surgery, but nurses do try to keep noise to a minimum.

What are the final preparations before an operation? I do rather dread the run-up to surgery.

You would be unusual if you didn't feel like this, but at least you'll know then that surgery will soon be over.

For an abdominal operation, your pubic hair needs to be shaved or removed with a depilatory cream (the hospital will provide the razor or cream). You will probably prefer to do this yourself, and it can be done before you take a bath or shower, but if you don't feel up to it a nurse will do it for you. You will also have to change into the gown (the opening goes at the back) and cap provided. No make-up or jewellery can be worn, but a nurse can put tape over any ring you prefer to leave on. Dentures or contact lenses must be removed. These preparations can be the most unnerving part, but the nurses will try to reassure you.

You will be given pre-medication either in the form of tablets or an injection into your buttock or thigh about an hour before surgery. This has a calming effect and will make you sleepy. It also dries up urine and saliva, which is why your mouth will be dry after the operation.

When it is time for the operation, you are lifted onto a trolley and a hospital porter will wheel you to the operating theatre. A nurse will also go with you and may hold your hand

and talk to you, which can be reassuring. The surgeon may greet you as you arrive at the operating theatre, although you probably won't remember much about all this afterwards. Just before you go into the operating theatre, the anaesthetist will inject the anaesthetic into a vein in the back of your hand. You will not be aware of anything after that.

I worry that my operation will go wrong — there are such frightening stories in the papers.

The chances of this happening to you are extremely remote, and certainly not worth worrying about before surgery. People very seldom actually die on the operating table. In the unlikely event of your operation going wrong in any way, or if you have any other complaint against the hospital, there is a complaints procedure; you can also take legal advice. But literally millions of operations are carried out safely each year; it is only the very few that go wrong which make headlines.

Will I be in pain after surgery?

As we said at the start of this chapter, you will be less sensitive to pain if you are calm and relaxed. Painkillers are in any case given whenever needed, and you have only to ask, so don't worry about this. In fact, you may find that the nurses ask you very frequently if you have any pain following surgery. Immediately after major surgery, painkillers may be given by injection into your buttock or thigh, or via a drip (see the next question). They can be taken by mouth within two days.

You must expect some discomfort, however. You may feel rather sick after recovering consciousness, and may be sick, although this is less usual with modern anaesthetics. If nausea is severe, you can be given an injection to quell it. You are also likely to be thirsty. You won't however be given anything to drink straight away, because this could make you sick, but you will be allowed sips of water or perhaps be given a piece of ice to suck. The digestive system tends to go on strike after surgery, due to the anaesthetic, so it may take a day or two before you are able to eat and drink.

In a very few hospitals the pain-relieving value of acupuncture* is being recognized; it can also relieve nausea. It is still unlikely that you will be offered this, but you may find it helpful when recovering at home. In any event, you should be over any severe pain before you leave hospital, and the nurses will do their best to make you comfortable.

In film dramas you see people who have had major surgery lying there full of tubes. How true to life is this?

You have to allow for dramatic effect in a film. In real life you may find yourself on a drip after a major operation. Don't be surprised or alarmed by this − it is simply used to replace fluid lost during surgery and because you cannot drink directly afterwards. The bag of fluid is attached to a stand by the bed; there is a tube from it leading to a needle which is inserted into a vein in the back of your hand or in your arm. This is painless.

Similarly, you may need a blood transfusion to replace blood lost during surgery, and this is given in the same way. It is also painless and over quite soon. The blood you are given will have been matched with your own (one reason why a blood sample would have been taken when you arrived in hospital). All blood is now tested for hepatitis and HIV (the virus that can cause AIDS), so there's no need to worry about infection from someone else's blood.

As already mentioned, painkillers can also be given by drip. You may therefore have two or three slim tubes taped to your hand or arm.

After a major abdominal or vaginal operation, such as a hysterectomy*, there may be a drain, i.e. a tube leading from the wound to remove any collection of fluid. It may be left there for a day or two and drains into a bottle or bag under the bed, or into an absorbent pad on your abdomen, which is changed as necessary.

A catheter can be needed to help you urinate. This is a slim tube inserted into your urethra which carries urine into a bag, which is also under the bed. Neither of these tubes is painful, although they may be just a little uncomfortable. If the catheter is needed for more than a day or two (as with operations involving the bladder), it may be placed in the bladder through the abdominal wall at the level of the pubic hairline. This may sound alarming, but in practice it is not. To remove it, the tube is gently pulled out; the bladder and abdominal wall heal naturally afterwards.

You will not necessarily require all, or any of this equipment after surgery. It depends on the operation you are having, so see the chapter on your particular condition.

How soon will I be mobile after major surgery, and how will I feel then? I don't like the thought of being helpless and undignified.

After a major operation you certainly won't be able to get out of bed unaided right away. You will also need to use a bedpan or commode to start with; this is easier if you are in a private room, but in a ward at least there is the consolation of knowing that you are not the only one who has to do this.

You will be encouraged to get up and walk around within a day or two, after the doctor or surgeon has checked you. Moving about is important because it prevents blood clots from forming in your legs as a result of being immobile in bed. You can still move around if you are on a drip or have a drain or catheter. It's simply a matter of carrying the equipment, and a nurse will help with this if necessary. You will also be encouraged to sit out of bed during the day.

You are likely to feel fragile and unsteady, but this feeling can be as much psychological as physical; surgery is a shock to the system.

When will my stitches be removed, and will this hurt?

Any incision will be covered by a dressing after surgery. A nurse will check this and may change it the next day. It will probably be removed within a couple of days. The wound will then be protected by either a fine plastic film, which is sprayed on, or – more usually – by an antibiotic spray. Stitches are removed in about five to seven days' time, so after a major operation this will be done before you leave hospital. Following a minor procedure, you will be sent home and the stitches will be taken out later by a doctor or nurse. Removal should not hurt if it is done carefully.

Soluble stitches are sometimes used; these do not need to be removed because they simply dissolve away. The type of stitch used depends on the operation you are having and on the surgeon's technique. Sometimes the incision is closed with metal clips, which a doctor or nurse can easily remove.

It is worth saying here that some women find it difficult to look at their incision – this is particularly true after breast surgery. Looking at it for the first time in a mirror may help, as this is less direct. You may be surprised at how neat it is.

Major surgery can have a deep emotional impact, and you will cope much better if you are prepared by counselling and reading this book.

Will I need to do any special exercises to help myself recover?

If necessary, a hospital physiotherapist will give you advice. For instance, abdominal and pelvic floor muscles can be weakened by surgery, and can be toned by doing certain exercises. There are also exercises which can help following breast surgery. See the chapter on your particular condition for more information.

I don't want to look a mess while I'm in hospital, especially when I have visitors. How can I avoid this?

You won't look your best immediately after surgery – and no one will expect you to. The nurses will wash you and comb your hair, if you are unable to do this yourself. But you will soon start to feel brighter and probably be able to do all these things for yourself within a couple of days. Hospitals often have hairdressing and manicure services, as either part of the hospital or on a hired-in basis, so you can take advantage of these. Nurses are aware that if you look nice you are likely to feel better too, and may help you with this.

How will I feel when I get home?

It is sensible to think about this beforehand. Hospitals provide a supportive environment which you will probably miss when you have to adjust to normal life again. Bear in mind that after an operation many women still feel very tired – or tire very easily – even though they are progressing physically. Specific advice on recovery is given in the chapters devoted to each particular condition.

The surgeon will want to check you, and you can also see your own doctor. These are opportunities to discuss any problems. You may find you need more help at home, in which case your doctor or the hospital social worker will be able to put you in touch with the right services.

It's not at all uncommon to feel depressed after returning home, and difficulties may arise in intimate relationships as a result of certain types of surgery. This is when counselling can be very helpful, as advised at the start of this chapter, so don't hesitate to ask for help if you feel you need it.

If you are having any further treatment following surgery, such as radiotherapy* and/or chemotherapy*, you may feel that 'it isn't over yet'. But further treatment should be viewed as promoting recovery. People who have a positive attitude and are determined to get well are actually helping themselves to do so, and this is where counselling and alternative therapies can also be very helpful.

Fortunately, many people look back on the time they spent in hospital as being very worthwhile, and feel the experience has increased their understanding of life.

3

RESOLVING PERIOD PROBLEMS

Increasingly, women with period problems can expect to be taken seriously and treated sympathetically. 'Monthly misery' is no longer seen as just a natural part of women's lot in life: the 'curse' which has to be endured. More is now known about the causes of period problems, and treatment with drugs and self-help methods can bring relief in many cases. But until quite recently surgery could offer little in the way of treatment. A woman suffering from that most debilitating of menstrual disorders – heavy and/or painful periods – could well find that a hysterectomy* to remove the womb was the only long-term solution. Now, however, this major operation is becoming less necessary for women with this problem. New minor surgical procedures, described as 'minimally invasive', are offering safe and speedy alternatives. Below we explain who can benefit from them and how they are carried out.

Why can't all women with heavy, painful periods be treated by the new surgical methods?

In order for these treatments to work, there must be little or no underlying disease. In other words, the womb (uterus) must be essentially normal, or if there are, for example, fibroids* (benign growths in the wall of the womb) causing the problem, they must be small. If the fibroids are large, or there is another underlying problem, such as endometriosis*, then different surgery is needed.

We must also make a distinction between heavy periods and painful periods: the two may go together, but not always. At the time of writing, these minimally invasive operations are being evaluated. Although they look very promising as treatments for heavy bleeding, it's less clear to what extent they will abolish period pains.

Who can benefit from the new surgical treatments?

A considerable number of women suffer from heavy, painful periods which may be due to an imbalance in the hormones produced during their menstrual cycle (see page 43). This tends to occur either in teenagers when periods first start, or when fertility is declining towards the menopause; this can happen to women in their mid- to late 30s onwards. The new treatments wouldn't be suitable for young women because afterwards it's virtually impossible to conceive. But for older women who have completed their families, the treatments can literally bring instant relief.

What are the treatments called, and how do they work?

They are called endometrial ablation and endometrial resection. The endometrium is the womb lining. Endometrial ablation permanently destroys the womb lining; either a powerful beam of laser light is used, or a 'microwave' tube is inserted into the uterus; the latter technique is called radiofrequency-induced endometrial ablation. With both methods, the heat generated achieves the result.

Endometrial resection removes the womb lining by cutting it away, so it does not grow back. The womb lining is shed each month (this is what a period is), so if it no longer exists, the problem of heavy periods will cease. If period pains are also a problem, they may disappear too. However, some women may still have pains each month, even when there is little or no bleeding.

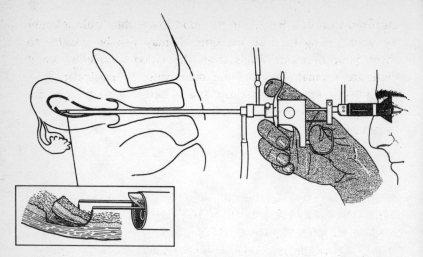

Endometrial resection removes the womb lining by cutting with a resectoscope, so treating heavy periods. Endometrial ablation achieves the same result using heat.

I feel exhausted all the time because of my heavy, painful periods. If I saw my doctor, would I be offered endometrial ablation or resection right away?

No, you would first be investigated to find the cause of your problem, for the reasons given in the first question (see page 36). Your doctor can refer you to a gynaecologist who will carry this investigation out.

The investigation would of course start with a routine pelvic examination* and, depending on what was found, might include an ultrasound scan*. Later, you may need a D & C (dilation and curettage)* or suction curettage*. These minor procedures are used to biopsy (remove) samples of womb lining for analysis. Sometimes a D & C can help improve heavy, painful periods, but tends not to be a successful long-term treatment; it's therefore used more often to find the cause of the problem. Finally, you may require a laparoscopy* (possibly combined with the D & C) so that the gynaecologist is able to get a direct look at your pelvic organs. This isn't to say that you will need all these procedures.

A blood test will show whether you are anaemic and suffering from iron deficiency due to blood loss – this could account for your feeling tired all the time. It may also be possible to check your hormone levels from the blood sample to see if these are normal. Towards the menopause in particular, hormone levels may indicate how much longer your periods are likely to continue, which could influence the decision to have treatment.

What would happen next?

Treatment usually starts with certain painkillers, taken in tablet form, which also have the effect of reducing bleeding. They are needed only during periods. If a hormone imbalance is diagnosed, you would most likely be given hormone treatment initially and iron supplements to help with anaemia. Should these fail to resolve the problem, then ablation or resection would be possible.

In some women, no specific cause can be found for their heavy, painful periods. Endometrial ablation/resection is likely to be particularly effective for them because, as mentioned earlier, the treatment is designed for women whose pelvic organs are normal.

If you are going to have laser or 'microwave' treatment, you would probably need to take a hormone drug for four to six weeks beforehand. This shrinks the womb lining so it is thinner and easier to ablate. Your periods may cease while you are on this drug. However, if you are having endometrial resection, it's not always essential to take hormones before the operation, although some surgeons do insist on it.

You say endometrial ablation and resection are minor procedures. How long would I be in hospital, and what would be done to me?

You would be in hospital for no more than a day – maybe even in before breakfast and out for supper. If you find yourself suffering from pre-op nerves, try to relax (see page 265 for advice on this); reading the rest of the chapter should also help to reassure you that this treatment is no big ordeal.

You are likely to be given a general anaesthetic, and therefore will be asked not to eat or drink for about four hours before surgery. However, some surgeons may give you a local anaesthetic instead. If so, it is helpful to know what to expect.

1. On arrival you would change into a surgical gown. It is not necessary for your pubic hair to be shaved. You are then given sedative tablets or an injection to help you relax and make you sleepy. After this, some women aren't aware of anything and don't remember what happens next; others are more awake, but still do not experience any pain.

2. In the operating theatre, your legs are supported apart by stirrups. The vaginal area is thoroughly cleaned with non-stinging antiseptic – although the inside of the vagina cannot be completely sterilized because it is always open to the air, in which bacteria (germs) are constantly floating. A local anaesthetic is then injected into the cervix (the entrance to the womb, also called the 'neck of the womb'). This hurts only momentarily.

3. The cervix is dilated (widened) using metal or plastic rods, and a hysteroscope*, a viewing instrument no thicker than a pencil, is inserted into the womb. It allows the surgeon a good view inside because it has a light and a telescopic lens.

4. Fluid is run into the womb and out again via the hysteroscope. This keeps the view clear during surgery.

5. How the procedure is then carried out depends on the surgeon's technique and the hospital's equipment, but here are the possible approaches:

   a) Endometrial ablation. This is done with a laser, as already mentioned, which is inserted via a channel in the hysteroscope. The powerful cutting beam of laser light burns the womb lining completely away and seals it at the same time so there is no bleeding. The whole procedure takes 15 to 30 minutes. The 'microwave' technique, also mentioned earlier, uses heat waves to destroy the womb lining, but at the time of writing is the procedure most seldom used.

b) Endometrial resection. For this a resectoscope is used. This instrument is similar to a hysteroscope, but in addition to the thin telescope, there is a small wire loop at the end. An electric current is passed through the wire loop, which is used to shave away the womb lining: the heat generated by the current both cuts the tissue and seals the blood vessels, preventing bleeding. Because you are 'earthed' by a pad on your thigh you won't feel the electricity passing through the wall of the womb. This procedure also takes 15 to 30 minutes.

The advantage of using a resectoscope is that the tissue can be sent for analysis under a microscope to ensure that no disease exists. This is not possible with laser treatment, because the womb lining is completely destroyed. You would therefore have a D & C beforehand to provide tissue for analysis, which isn't always necessary prior to a resection.

Is that the end of the treatment?

Yes. You will spend several hours in the recovery room resting until the sedative or anaesthetic wears off, and then you can go home. Before you leave hospital your blood-pressure is checked and you will be given painkillers to take if necessary. Pain is usually minimal; you may also experience slight bleeding. Arrange for someone to take you home because you may be feeling a bit shaky, although this is more of a psychological than physical reaction. You certainly should not drive.

Are there any after-effects? How long does recovery take?

There are unlikely to be any after-effects. You may be advised to take things easy for about a week, but many women often feel back to normal in a day or two. Expect to have a blood-stained, watery discharge for between one and four weeks; this is normal. If, however, the discharge has an offensive odour, this may mean you have an infection. This wouldn't be due to medical negligence; it is just that the vagina is never a sterile environment. Consult your doctor, who can prescribe antibiotics. Use sanitary towels and not tampons, because tampons encourage infection. Don't have sex until the discharge ceases. Showering or bathing is safe from day one. Usually all that is then needed is a formal check with your surgeon after six weeks, to ensure that all is well.

Will I ever have periods again after endometrial ablation or resection?

At the time of writing, it would seem that at least 90 per cent of women do not have periods, or have only slight bleeding, after these procedures.

Do I still need to use contraception?

Yes. Even though the chances of your becoming pregnant after surgery are extremely remote, it's still advisable to go on using contraception, just in case. Your doctor will advise you on how long this should continue.

How much better are these techniques than having a hysterectomy* to resolve heavy bleeding?

A hysterectomy involves major abdominal surgery to remove the entire womb, a stay of 7 to 14 days in hospital, and several months convalescence. In addition there is the emotional trauma experienced by some women at losing a part of themselves which they value highly. The difference is that endometrial ablation and resection involve none of these things, yet achieve practically the same result – with minimal inconvenience to a woman. They are becoming increasingly available in hospitals. Comments from women who have been treated include 'absolutely fantastic' and 'I couldn't believe how simple it was.'

Questions Women Most Often Ask About Resolving Period Problems

You said earlier that a hormone imbalance is often responsible for heavy periods. How does this happen?

There is a detailed description of how hormones control the menstrual cycle in Chapter 4. Briefly, heavy periods, which may be painful, can often be related to an imbalance in the two hormones produced by the ovaries, namely oestrogen and progesterone. These prepare the womb lining for a pregnancy. Oestrogen does this during the first part of the menstrual cycle, prior to ovulation* (the release of a ripe egg). After ovulation, both hormones further prepare the womb to receive a fertilized egg. If there is no pregnancy, the womb lining is shed as a period. Heavy periods can occur when there is too much oestrogen or too little progesterone. This means that the womb lining goes on growing and is shed as a heavy period, although not necessarily on a regular monthly basis. Often the menstrual cycle is irregular. This may happen because ovulation isn't taking place (although scanty, irregular periods can also be a sign of this; it depends on the level of oestrogen).

In young girls, ovulation may not occur simply because periods can begin before regular ovulation gets under way. This usually resolves itself, or can be helped by hormone treatment. In older women, as already stated, the natural decline in fertility may be responsible, and hormone treatment does not always work. Stress can also influence our hormones.

Earlier you mentioned self-help methods of dealing with period problems. What are these?

If there is no underlying disease causing the problem, simple, well-tried methods, such as taking aspirin or paracetamol and holding a hot water bottle to the abdomen, can bring temporary relief from menstrual pain. Some women find that a balanced diet, relaxation techniques, Yoga, massage, hypnosis or acupuncture have all helped improve the problem of heavy, painful periods (see Chapter 18 on Alternative Therapies and Healthier Living).

An area of the brain called the hypothalamus co-ordinates our nervous and hormonal systems; it also registers our emotions, which could be why stress, anxiety and unhappiness may be associated with menstrual problems. But don't therefore feel that any such problems must somehow be your fault. As said earlier, sometimes there is no obvious cause. You should always see your doctor if you feel you need help.

4

INVESTIGATING AND TREATING INFERTILITY

Finding that you cannot conceive a much-wanted child is one of the most distressing situations a woman and her partner can face. Fortunately, much can be done to investigate and treat female infertility; this chapter explains its possible causes, and advises on the tests and procedures which may be recommended to you. What must be emphasized is that this is a shared problem, so your partner's co-operation is essential. Very often, however, it is the woman who first seeks help.

I've been trying to become pregnant for some months now without success. Does this mean that one or both of us is infertile?

No, it can take time to conceive. Provided your periods are normal, and you are both in good health, many doctors would consider that you should try for at least a year before becoming concerned. If you are in your 20s, two years may be advised. A woman's fertility declines with age, as does a man's, but in women this starts earlier. It may be more difficult to conceive once you are in your 30s, and by the mid-40s relatively few women become pregnant. So, if you are in your mid-30s, for example, it's sensible to seek help sooner rather than later.

Finding out why fertilization doesn't take place, and treating the problem, can be a lengthy process. Patience and perseverance may be needed, although some couples conceive quite quickly after starting treatment.

Where should I go for help?

Your own doctor or family planning clinic are the best sources of help to start with. The initial investigations may be carried out at this stage, or you may be referred directly to a gynaecologist or a specialist clinic. If possible your partner should go with you.

My partner is reluctant to become involved in fertility investigations.

This is often because men confuse fertility with virility. They may have the idea that being unable to father a child must somehow be connected with impotence – an inability to perform sexually. While this may sometimes be the problem, a man can have a satisfying sexual relationship and be infertile: the two can be quite separate. There would be no point in your having exhaustive investigations when the problem might be with your partner. If you both know what happens in fertilization, it will be easier to understand what might be wrong and how any tests or treatments proposed may help.

Could you explain how fertilization takes place?

Fertilization depends firstly on your producing a ripe egg during your menstrual cycle. This is controlled by hormones (which act as chemical messengers). They are produced by a gland located in the base of the brain, called the pituitary gland.

    At the start of a period – day one of your cycle – the pituitary releases a hormone called follicle stimulating hormone (FSH) which, as its name suggests, stimulates one of your ovaries to produce a follicle. This looks like a small capsule on the surface of the ovary, and it contains a developing egg (ovum). During the next 12 to 14 days, the follicle and egg ripen. At the same time, the ovary produces a hormone called oestrogen; this prepares the womb (uterus) for a pregnancy. Mucus secretions from the cervix (the entrance to the womb) are thick, cloudy and sticky at this stage.

    Next the pituitary produces luteinizing hormone (LH) in

response to the oestrogen. LH causes the follicle to burst and release the ripe egg, on about day 14. This is ovulation. The follicle then forms yellow tissue, called the corpus luteum or 'yellow body', which secretes the hormone progesterone. There is usually a small drop in body temperature and then a rise of about $0.6°C/1°F$ caused by the progesterone, which shows that ovulation has occurred. You won't be aware of the change in temperature, although some women do feel a little abdominal pain at ovulation and may have a pinkish vaginal discharge.

What happens after ovulation?

The egg is scooped up by the fronds (fimbriae) located at the end of the Fallopian tube near the ovary, enabling the egg to enter the tube. This is where fertilization takes place. Cervical mucus is now thinner, stringier and wetter, to allow your partner's sperm to swim from the vagina, up the cervix, through the womb and into the tube. One sperm penetrates the egg and fertilizes it.

Fertilization therefore also depends on your partner producing enough healthy, mobile sperm and ejaculating them high enough in the vagina at the right time.

After fertilization, the egg develops for about three days in the Fallopian tube. Meanwhile, oestrogen and progesterone further prepare the womb, the egg travels there, implants in the lining, and becomes a pregnancy. If fertilization does not take place, hormone levels drop and the womb lining is shed as a period on about day 28. The cycle then begins again.

Although this description is based on an average 28-day cycle, variations in the number of days in any woman's cycle are not uncommon or abnormal. However, you are most likely to be fertile around the middle of your cycle, and therefore to have the best chance of conceiving then, provided there are no problems.

How will the doctor go about finding out what might be wrong?

You and your partner will be interviewed separately and together, and be asked a wide range of questions. Be prepared to be completely open and honest about your sex life, and about your medical history, if this isn't already known. This information is essential; the doctor will most likely proceed in a tactful and sensitive manner, to minimize any embarrassment.

What sort of questions will I be asked?

The doctor is likely to ask you:

- about your periods and menstrual pattern
- when and how often you have sex
- what contraception you have used
- if you have ever been pregnant, and if so, by whom. What happened to the pregnancy, e.g. termination*, miscarriage*, ectopic pregnancy*, live birth? This may reveal why you are having problems now
- whether you've had any sexually transmitted diseases (STDs)
- if you've ever had abdominal surgery
- what you and your partner's lifestyle is like, i.e. how much attention you pay to diet, exercise, relaxation – all of which can affect fertility (see page 65)

Will we be examined?

Yes, certainly. Routine physical examinations are carried out to check the general health of both partners and to see if there are any obvious problems which could affect conception. You will be given a pelvic examination* and your partner's genitals will also need to be examined.

What is the next step?

This depends on the doctor's assessment of your situation. As already mentioned, with some couples sexual performance may be the problem – and this can apply to either partner. For instance, the man may have erection difficulties, or the woman be reluctant to have sex. The causes could be physical or psychological. Medical treatment or psychosexual therapy is often successful, and the doctor would refer the couple for the necessary help.

Occasionally, even today, not being fully informed about the facts of life is the problem, and a simple explanation the solution.

Assuming there are no such difficulties in your case, nor any other obvious problems which need medical attention, then the doctor may discuss a treatment plan with you. It must be stressed, however, that you won't necessarily proceed from one test or treatment to the next; a number of different approaches may need to be tried. You may be advised to take your temperature every morning immediately on waking (using an ordinary oral thermometer) and record it on a special chart for about three months. This may show whether you are ovulating; the dip and rise in temperature is the sign. It may also be helpful if you check the state of your cervical mucus. Having intercourse at the time of ovulation is of course essential, and so you may also be asked to record when you have sex on the chart.

Will my partner be investigated at this stage?

Yes. He will be asked not to ejaculate for three days (this can maximize the number of sperm), and then provide a sample of semen by masturbating into a clean jar, warmed to body temperature. The semen will be analysed to find out the proportion of sperm in it (this is called a sperm count) and whether or not they are properly shaped and mobile. A minimum of 20 to 25 million sperm per ml of semen is considered necessary for fertilization, and usually the count is higher than this. 75 per cent should look normal and be moving around. If his sperm count is low, the test may be repeated two or three times (at intervals), because the count can vary. He may also be advised not to ejaculate for three days before having intercourse at the crucial time, as this may make conception more likely. The first part of the ejaculation may contain more sperm, and so withdrawing the penis from the vagina before ejaculation is complete may also increase the chances of conception. Although a consistently low sperm count is often associated with infertility, it doesn't always mean a man can't father a child. A very low count or a complete absence of sperm, however, does need further investigation.

Are there any further preliminary tests?

Some doctors may want to carry out post-coital and/or sperm invasion tests. These show how your partner's sperm behave when they come into contact with your cervical mucus.

The post-coital test requires you to have intercourse around the time of ovulation and then visit the doctor either the next morning or within a few hours, without disturbing the vagina by washing or douching.

As in a routine pelvic examination*, your vagina will be opened with a speculum and a small amount of mucus sucked from the cervix by syringe or pipette. This causes little discomfort. The sample is placed on a glass slide and examined through a microscope. It should show healthy sperm swimming actively in thin, stretchy mucus. Sperm should be able to survive inside a woman for at least 48 hours. Dead sperm and sperm marooned in thick, sticky mucus indicate problems.

The mucus may be too thick for penetration, or there may be too little to allow sperm to swim to the cervix; or the sperm may be having trouble surviving because the mucus is 'hostile' – i.e. it contains antibodies to them, which creates a reaction similar to an allergy; or there may be a problem with the sperm themselves. A man can form antibodies to his own sperm which kill them. No one knows why antibody problems occur.

How does the sperm invasion test help?

This more recent test can help to determine whether the problem is due to the sperm or mucus. You don't need to have intercourse beforehand. Some mucus is removed from the vagina, as already described, and placed on a slide, together with a small sample of your partner's semen. The sperm should swim easily into the mucus, but if the mucus is 'hostile' it will cause the sperm to quiver, clump together and die. Donor sperm from a man known to be fertile can also be introduced to your mucus on a slide to see if they can penetrate it. This is called a cross-over sperm invasion test.

What can be done to resolve mucus problems?

Treating the woman with oestrogen hormones in the first half of her menstrual cycle can sometimes resolve mucus penetration problems. If there is a mild vaginal infection, such as thrush, which may be slowing down the sperm, this can also be treated. Dealing with antibodies can be more difficult as they don't always respond to drug treatment, but there are techniques for overcoming this problem, described later in this chapter.

Three months seems a long time for these preliminary investigations.

This allows time for both partners' fertility to be assessed, so that the doctor can decide how to proceed. Couples sometimes achieve a pregnancy during this time anyway. If not, this period of time also tests their resolve to pursue treatment, which – as already said – may be lengthy and demanding. Partners who keep up the daily temperature charts, and have sex when conception is most likely, would be seen as more suitable candidates for further treatment than those who are less determined.

What other investigations might we need?

If the problem appears to be with your partner, see page 59. However, it may turn out to be shared problem, such as a low sperm count combined with a lack of ovulation; or the problem may be entirely with you. More can be done to investigate and treat female infertility than male. This isn't meant to discourage partners where the man has a problem; it's simply that there are currently more approaches to female problems, and so these are covered next.

Is failure to ovulate one of the most common reasons for female infertility?

Yes, which is why investigations often start with this aspect if no other problems are apparent.

Why would a woman fail to ovulate?

Frequently it is due to an imbalance in the hormones responsible. Irregular, scanty or missed periods are often a sign of this. Ovarian tumours* or the condition known as polycystic ovaries* (where there are numerous small cysts) can prevent ovulation. It may result from discontinuing the pill, which acts by altering hormone levels to suppress ovulation. Usually hormone levels readjust quite quickly after discontinuing the pill, but occasionally there is a problem.

Sometimes there is no obvious reason. Stress may play a part in reducing fertility in both men and women (more on this later), but there needs to be a thorough medical investigation before this is considered a possibility.

How are the causes diagnosed?

Keeping temperature charts can be a useful initial guide to whether ovulation is occurring, but is not entirely reliable. Some of the following may be tried.

- Tests on blood and urine made in the second half of the menstrual cycle will show if there is a hormonal imbalance. There are home urine testing kits available, but these are more useful for fertile women who want to pinpoint ovulation than for those who may have fertility problems.
- An endometrial biopsy* (removal of a sample of womb lining) carried out at the time ovulation should occur will also uncover a hormonal imbalance. This can be done under local or general anaesthetic – see D & C (dilation and curettage)* and suction curettage*.
- The ovaries can be viewed by ultrasound*; or they can be

directly seen by laparoscopy*, which is carried out under general anaesthetic at a hospital or clinic.

- An X-ray* of the pituitary gland can be taken, to see if it appears normal.

What treatments are there for these problems?

Hormonal problems can often be treated successfully with fertility drugs; they can also restart ovulation if necessary after the pill has been discontinued. Polycystic ovaries* may also respond to drug treatment, but sometimes surgery is needed. Ovarian tumours* may need surgery too.

Are there any other causes of female infertility?

Other major causes are blocked or scarred Fallopian tubes and adhesions (scar tissue) in the pelvis. Damaged tubes prevent sperm and egg from meeting, or can cause a fertilized egg to lodge in a tube; this is called an ectopic pregnancy*. An ectopic pregnancy has to be removed by surgery, and sometimes the Fallopian tube also. Adhesions can gum up and distort the tubes and bind the pelvic organs together so they can't move freely, as is necessary for conception.

Why do tubal problems and adhesions occur?

Blocked or scarred Fallopian tubes most often result from inflammation (called salpingitis) due to infection. Untreated gonorrhoea and chlamydia are common causes. These are transmitted during unprotected intercourse with an infected person. Practically everyone these days must know how essential condoms are for avoiding HIV. They are just as vital in preventing the spread of these fertility-threatening sexually transmitted diseases (STDs), which are particularly dangerous because for women the symptoms seldom develop until the infection is advanced. By then, adhesions and abscesses may have formed on the tubes and ovaries.

An infected woman will eventually experience unpleasant

symptoms such as painful irregular periods, abdominal cramps, backache, fever, fatigue and a brown or yellowish foul-smelling discharge. In addition, adhesions can make sex painful when pressure is put on them during intercourse. Pelvic inflammatory disease (PID) is the name given to this very serious condition.

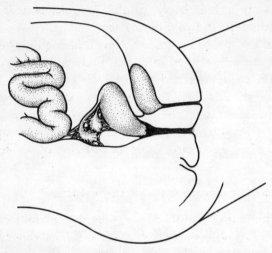

Adhesions which block and distort the Fallopian tubes are a major cause of infertility. They can sometimes be freed using laser or microsurgical techniques.

Sexual behaviour is not the only cause of PID; it can be due to infection following termination*, miscarriage* or childbirth, although better procedures have made this much less usual nowadays.

Do these problems have any other causes?

Yes, adhesions and other problems can be caused by endometriosis. This disorder tends to affect childless women over the age of 30, although occasionally it occurs in younger, usually childless, women. It happens because pieces of the endometrium (womb lining) are present outside the womb; they may be in the muscular wall of the womb, on the peritoneum (the lining of the pelvic cavity), on the tubes and ovaries, or on other organs, such as the bowel or bladder. These pieces of the endometrium respond to the hormonal changes of the menstrual cycle by bleeding during periods. This results in inflammation, to which the body reacts by forming scar tissue around the pieces. Sometimes blood-filled 'chocolate' cysts (so-called because their contents resemble chocolate sauce) form on the ovaries and may grow to the size of oranges. Symptoms can include heavy, painful, irregular periods, chronic pelvic discomfort, and pain during sex.

Why endometriosis occurs is unclear. Although it often causes infertility, not all women with the problem are infertile – it depends on the position and extent of the stray tissue.

Other causes of adhesions include peritonitis – inflammation of the peritoneum – which may result from a ruptured appendix. They can also form after an abdominal operation, which may have been carried out for this kind of problem.

If these disorders are suspected, how would they be diagnosed?

- **Laparoscopy*** is used to diagnose both endometriosis and PID. Any damage can be assessed by viewing the pelvic organs directly through the laparoscope; this is usually done under general anaesthetic. A test can be carried out during the procedure to discover the state of the tubes: a harmless dye is injected into the womb through a tube inserted into the cervix, and the laparoscope used to see if the dye emerges from the tubes (see illustration on page 16) – any blockage would prevent this. Afterwards you would have a dye-coloured vaginal discharge for a few days and would need to use sanitary towels. You would also have the usual minor discomfort following any laparoscopy, but would recover quickly.
- **Hysterosalpingography** (HSG) is a test which finds out where the tube is blocked. It may be performed after laparoscopy has shown there is a blockage. HSG also involves injecting dye into the womb, via a slim tube inserted in the cervix. The dye is radio-opaque, which means that the inside of the womb and Fallopian tubes will show on an X-ray*. The whole procedure takes from 10 to 30 minutes and is done on an out-patient basis. An

anaesthetic is not usually used, but you may be given a sedative injection because the procedure can be uncomfortable, causing menstrual-type cramps. You may need a day to recover and, again, will have a dye-coloured discharge.

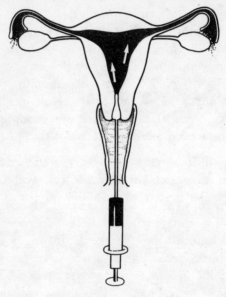

(1) In a hysterosalpingogram (HSG) harmless dye, which can be seen by X-ray, is injected into the womb and Fallopian tubes.

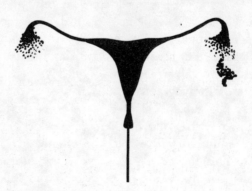

(2) An X-ray of normal tubes releasing the dye.

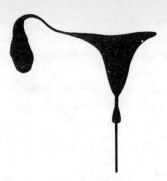

(3) *An X-ray of damaged tubes — on the right the dye has been blocked near the womb; on the left the tube has become sac-like and swollen with fluid.*

Are there any treatments to overcome these disorders?

Yes, although their success cannot be guaranteed; much depends on the type and extent of the problem. For instance, pelvic infections can be treated with antibiotics, but this won't clear up adhesions or tubal damage caused by severe PID. Similarly, endometriosis responds to drugs which prevent ovulation and menstruation, so the affected areas shrink and, if small, may disappear. However, large areas, chocolate cysts or adhesions cannot be treated this way. Surgery may be helpful in restoring fertility, but it has to be said that severe widespread endometriosis or PID may necessitate a hysterectomy*, which would end fertility. This should always be the treatment of last resort, especially if the woman is of childbearing age.

What kind of surgery may help restore fertility?

It may be possible to carry out laser surgery with a laparoscope. This uses a high-energy beam of light for cutting, which also prevents bleeding and avoids damage to surrounding tissue. Adhesions can be separated, freeing the pelvic organs, and patches of endometriosis burnt off. If a tubal blockage is located at the end of the tube near the ovary, the tube can sometimes be opened up and the fimbriae freed. As with all laparoscopy procedures, surgery is carried out in hospital under general anaesthetic, but you will only be in for a day or two. You may have some internal soreness afterwards and need painkillers, but will be able to resume normal life quite quickly; there is no need to convalesce.

If the problem is more extensive, then the abdomen would need to be opened for surgery using a procedure called a laparotomy. This may follow straight on from an investigation by laparoscopy, and you would therefore remain unconscious between procedures. You would of course be asked to sign a consent form before the laparoscopy, and must be sure you understand what a laparotomy entails.

How is a laparotomy carried out?

An incision measuring about 10 cm (4 in) is made in the lower abdomen across the pubic hairline, although a larger incision up the abdomen is sometimes necessary – the surgeon will endeavour to keep it to the minimum.

Fine microsurgical instruments are used to divide adhesions and to remove cysts and endometriosis. Sometimes blocked Fallopian tubes can be reconstructed by cutting out the blocked section and joining the ends together, but as each tube is just 7.5 cm (3 in) long only a small section can be removed. Surgery cannot restore tubes which have become severely blocked and swollen with fluid.

This is a major operation, and it will help you to read Chapter 2 on Preparing for Surgery. Advice on your hospital stay (which will be for about a week) and on recovery is given in Chapter 12 on Ovarian Tumours, as they require similarly major surgery.

If you've had one or both tubes unblocked, they may need 'washing through' to keep them open in the days afterwards. This can be done by injecting fluid through the cervix, as for an HSG, or sometimes via a fine polythene tube brought out through the abdominal wall.

What are my chances of becoming pregnant after surgery?

It's not easy to predict how likely a particular woman is to conceive following surgery. Much depends on the severity of the problems and what needs to be done. Overall, the chances of success are around 15 to 30 per cent. But there is always the risk of an ectopic pregnancy* following tubal surgery. Also, it has to said that surgery to remove adhesions may itself cause more to form.

When can I try for a baby?

If you've had endometriosis removed, you may still be advised to take drugs which prevent ovulation for a few months afterwards − to shrink any remaining areas and ensure the best chance of success. You would not be able to become pregnant until treatment was discontinued. Following other surgery, you can usually restart intercourse after your post-operative check-up six weeks later, but if you've had a laparotomy, you may need to wait three to six months to recover fully before trying to conceive. Your doctor will advise you.

If my partner has fertility problems, how can he be helped?

Where a man's sperm count is consistently very low, or there are no sperm, he would probably be referred to an andrologist (a specialist in problems of the male reproductive system). Often this work is also covered by a urologist (a specialist in urinary tract disorders) who has a particular interest in male infertility. The major causes of male infertility would be investigated and tests done to find out whether any of the following problems are present:

- the seminal vesicles (the sperm-carrying tubes) in the scrotum are blocked by infection from untreated STDs;
- there is a prostate infection. This gland at the base of the penis produces seminal fluid; an infection can be toxic to sperm and make them less mobile;

- there is a varicocele (like a varicose vein) in the scrotum. This would raise the temperature of the scrotum, and heat inhibits sperm production;
- a hormonal imbalance is responsible.

Treatment can be as follows:

- antibiotics to clear STDs and prostatic infection;
- surgery to remove a varicocele (relatively simple, but with variable results), or to unblock tubes (probably less successful);
- hormone treatment to correct an imbalance (less successful than in women).

Smoking and excessive alcohol can make sperm less mobile, so drinking moderately and giving up smoking, or at least cutting down, may improve fertility.

Unfortunately, however, if a man's sperm production is totally defective, or if his tubes are irreversibly blocked, there is little chance of helping him. But for the man with impaired fertility, research is going on into ways of 'enhancing' sperm to free them of antibodies, or to pick out the most healthy sperm in a low sperm count. They can then be used in the techniques described on pages 61–5.

Why has my partner been advised to keep his genitals cool?

As already mentioned, heat is an enemy of sperm production. If there are no obvious problems which can be treated, 'DIY' methods of boosting fertility may help. If he avoids wallowing in hot baths or saunas, soaks his genitals daily in cold water, and wears loose underpants, his sperm count may improve.

My partner and I have had fertility investigations and there seems to be nothing wrong with us. Why can't we conceive?

There are cases of 'unexplained' infertility. It may help you to follow the advice given later about lifestyle and relaxation. But if this situation persists, the techniques described next may help.

Supposing there are fertility problems which can't be overcome by the treatments you have described, what can be done then?

Techniques of 'assisted conception' can sometimes get round the difficulties, although the success rate varies.

Artificial Insemination

Artificial insemination is a simple technique which maximizes the chances of conception by placing sperm directly inside the cervix. The woman's reproductive tract needs to be normal for this technique to be used.

WHY IT IS NEEDED
It is particularly helpful when the man has penetration problems which cannot be resolved, but is still fertile and can ejaculate. It is also helpful if his sperm count is low: the 'sperm rich' first part of the ejaculate can be used, and the sperm are given a better start. This technique also virtually bypasses 'hostile' mucus.

AIH (artificial insemination by husband) is the name given to the technique when your regular partner's sperm is used. But if his sperm count is very low, or non-existent, donor sperm from a fertile man can be used instead.

AID (artificial insemination by donor) requires careful thought and counselling beforehand, and the couple must be certain that a child conceived in this way is what they both want. If they decide to go ahead, a donor will be selected by the clinic in consultation with the couple. All donors are screened for hepatitis and HIV/AIDS, so there is no cause for concern about this.

HOW IT IS CARRIED OUT
For AIH, you and your partner visit the clinic at your fertile time (ovulation can be stimulated by fertility drugs if necessary). Your partner provides a semen sample, or a sample of his

which has been previously frozen by the clinic can be used. For the procedure, you lie on your back with your hips raised. A slim tube attached to a syringe containing the semen is inserted into your cervix and the semen introduced. It is painless and no anaesthetic is needed. Your partner can be with you throughout.

Previously frozen donor sperm is used in the same way for AID and, if you have chosen this option, your partner's presence can make it a shared experience.

Afterwards, you need to stay in the same position for about 30 minutes, or a cap can be fitted over the cervix so you can go home right away. The cap needs to be left in place for about eight hours.

The procedure may be carried out two or three times more during the fertile few days, and be repeated at the same time for up to six months if a pregnancy doesn't occur before then.

SUCCESS RATE

It is most successful when both partners are fertile and fresh semen is used. The success rate over six months is around 55 per cent when frozen semen is used; with fresh semen it is as high as 70 per cent.

In Vitro Fertilization (IVF)

IVF can overcome difficulties in bringing sperm and egg together by achieving fertilization outside the body. In vitro means 'in glass', which is where it takes place. This is why a child conceived in this way is called a 'test-tube baby', although a glass dish is actually used.

WHY IT IS NEEDED

When both of the woman's Fallopian tubes are irreversibly blocked or have been surgically removed due to ectopic pregnancies*, IVF can be tried, provided her ovaries and womb are healthy. It can sometimes succeed when the man's sperm count is low, particularly if his healthiest sperm are selected for use. Mucus 'hostility' can also be overcome by this technique.

HOW IT IS CARRIED OUT

Fertility drugs are given in the first part of the menstrual cycle (days 1 to 9), causing several egg follicles to ripen. Their progress is monitored by ultrasound* (days 10 to 13). Just prior to ovulation, further drugs may be given to complete ripening; the eggs are then 'harvested' before they are released from their follicles (days 14 to 6). This can be done in one of two ways.

1. The original technique uses laparoscopy* to see inside the pelvis. This requires a general anaesthetic and a stay of a day or two at the clinic. A fine hollow needle is inserted through the lower abdomen and used to suck the eggs from their follicles.

2. A more recent method uses a vaginal ultrasound probe. This is placed in the vagina so that the ovaries can be viewed. A fine needle at the tip of the probe is passed through the top of the vagina into the ovary to collect the ripe eggs. The procedure takes only a few minutes, and you will be given a local anaesthetic.

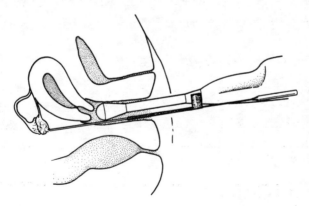

Ripe eggs being 'harvested' from the ovaries prior to in vitro fertilization (IVF). The ovaries are viewed via an ultrasound probe and a hollow needle passed through the top of the vagina to collect the eggs.

After the eggs are removed they are mixed with your partner's sperm in a glass dish and incubated for about 40 hours to bring about fertilization. Incubation can be done in a laboratory, but a more recent method is to incubate the mixture in a small tube placed in your vagina. It stays there just like a tampon and should not cause you any discomfort.

Up to three fertilized eggs (called embryos) are then placed in the womb via a slim tube inserted in the cervix; this requires no anaesthetic. Hopefully, at least one will implant and become a pregnancy. If conception takes place, there is an increased possibility of twins being conceived. There is no increased risk of birth defects of disorders, provided that not more than three embryos are inserted.

Remaining embryos not inserted into the womb can be frozen for future use if the first attempt fails. IVF has also been carried out on frozen eggs, i.e. eggs that have been removed to be fertilized at a later date. This resolves some of the ethical issues associated with frozen embryos.

SUCCESS RATE
About one in ten couples who try IVF will have a baby. Miscarriage* is a problem, and the older the woman, the less the chance of success; IVF may not always be considered for women over 40. However, it has made having a baby possible for women who would otherwise have had no chance whatsoever.

Gamete Intra-Fallopian Transfer (GIFT)

GIFT brings sperm and egg together for fertilization inside the woman's Fallopian tubes in a more natural way, gamete being the medical name used to describe both sperm and egg.

WHY IT IS NEEDED
GIFT is sometimes helpful if the woman's reproductive system is normal yet the couple have unexplained infertility. It also avoids the problem of 'hostile' mucus.

HOW IT IS CARRIED OUT
As with IVF, the ovaries are first stimulated with fertility drugs to produce ripe eggs. These eggs are then harvested by laparoscopy

under general anaesthetic. But, instead of fertilization taking place in a dish, about four eggs are mixed with sperm and put in the open ends of the Fallopian tubes (two in each tube), via the laparoscope, to enable fertilization to take place.

SUCCESS RATE

Around 30 per cent of couples who try GIFT achieve a pregnancy, but there is an increased risk of ectopic* and multiple pregnancies, although the technique is new at the time of writing and the risk has not been fully assessed.

Questions Women Most Often Ask About Infertility

How does one's lifestyle affect fertility?

It's particularly important for you both to be in the best possible health when you are trying to conceive. Your fertility can be impaired if you are very underweight or overweight, drink too much or smoke, or are under stress. All these factors can alter hormone levels. Try to eat sensibly and drink moderately, take regular exercise, and don't smoke (or at least try to cut down). Adequate rest and relaxation are essential, too. Your doctor will certainly advise you to adopt a healthier lifestyle, if necessary, and this may be all that is needed to enable you to conceive. Don't try to be super-fit, though. Excessive training can reduce fertility, as some athletes have found. See Chapter 18 for more information on healthier living.

It's all very well to say we should reduce stress, but fertility problems and treatment are a cause of it! What are we supposed to do about this?

The first thing to do is to think positively. By seeking help you have made a big step towards overcoming infertility. This in itself can help you relax. Alternative therapies may also help, such as Yoga, meditation, visualization, hypnosis and acupuncture (see Chapter 18).

Having intercourse 'to order' is proving very difficult.

Performing to order can be a turn-off; lovemaking becomes baby-making rather than a spontaneous pleasure. Try to relax, as advised above. Also try turning yourselves on at the crucial time. What turned you on before? The right atmosphere? Romantic meals? Reading erotica? Sex toys? Fantasy and romance? Concentrate on recreating that mood. The sex manuals listed in the References and Further Reading section may help.

Are there any positions for intercourse that help conception?

The man-on-top (or so-called 'missionary') position, with your hips raised on pillows, may help conception. Stay in this position for 15 minutes after your partner has ejaculated, to give the sperm the best chance of entering your cervix. But any sexual position which allows deep penetration favours conception, particularly if it's pleasurable and encourages you to make love.

Does it make conception more likely if the woman has an orgasm?

Some experts think it may help, but it's not essential. The point is to enjoy sex, and keep trying.

I've been told I have a retroverted womb. Will this make me less fertile?

No. About 20 per cent of women have a womb which is retroverted, i.e. tilted backwards instead of forwards in the pelvis. There is no evidence that this affects conception, unless it is held there rigidly by scar tissue. Treatment is then needed.

I have fibroids*. Is this why I can't conceive?

These benign growths in the muscular wall of the womb are not often a cause of infertility. If they are very large, however, or distort the cavity of the womb, a fertilized egg won't be able to implant. An operation called a myomectomy* can put this right. Similarly, a malformed womb may be unable to support a pregnancy; surgery can sometimes correct this.

Is the IUCD a cause of infertility?

Usually not. An IUCD (intra-uterine contraceptive device) is inserted in the womb and acts by slightly irritating the lining. This prevents a fertilized egg from implanting, and might delay pregnancy even when the device has been removed. It may also cause mild inflammation of the Fallopian tubes and thereby increase the risk of an ectopic pregnancy*. And if there is any infection, it may enter the reproductive tract more easily when an IUCD is in place. For all these reasons, women who have not had children and who wish to become pregnant later are generally advised not to use it.

We are having treatment for infertility, and feel very isolated by our problem. How can we cope?

Considerable emotional support is often needed to cope with fertility problems and their treatment. One is surrounded by families and perhaps under pressure from parents who want grandchildren. Feelings of isolation, and even failure, are quite natural. But you are not alone. Around one in six of all couples find they need specialist help at some time. There are support groups where you can meet others in your situation. Your doctor or fertility clinic can put you in touch with one.

How long is it realistic to go on being treated for infertility?

Only your doctor can advise you on this. Sometimes it may continue over several years. If every appropriate treatment is tried without success, the possibility of being permanently childless may have to be faced. This can be a profound test of a relationship, and requires a major adjustment. It is worth seeing a counsellor if you need help – ask your doctor about this. However, about 50 per cent of couples treated do achieve a pregnancy.

Is surrogacy an alternative?

Surrogacy is an arrangement whereby another woman agrees to bear a child for an infertile woman. In cases where the husband is fertile his sperm is used, with conception taking place either through intercourse (if this is acceptable to everyone involved), artificial insemination or in vitro fertilization. If both partners are fertile, but the woman has had her womb removed by hysterectomy*, leaving her ovaries intact, their child can be conceived by IVF. The fertilized egg could be implanted into the womb of a surrogate, who bears a child which is biologically that of both parents.

In some countries surrogacy is illegal; in others it is legal only if no money is involved. It is fraught with moral and practical dilemmas which have yet to be resolved. There have been tragic cases of surrogate mothers refusing to part with the child once it is born. It is therefore not a viable alternative for most infertile couples. Fostering or adoption are more acceptable solutions.

Does medical progress hold out greater hope to infertile couples?

Yes, definitely. Research into new techniques is continuing all the time, while existing treatments are being improved.

5

PROCEDURES IN PREGNANCY AND CHILDBIRTH

You're expecting a baby, and are looking forward to a fulfilling experience in pregnancy and childbirth. Nowadays women can feel more confident about giving birth: doctors may take a much more positive approach to natural childbirth, which gives mothers greater involvement and control. Medical intervention can, however, be helpful – and sometimes essential – during both pregnancy and childbirth, to detect and prevent any problems. In this chapter we explain the main diagnostic and surgical procedures which may be used, and why they can be necessary.

Diagnostic Procedures in Pregnancy

Why are diagnostic procedures offered in pregnancy?

All parents want a normal, healthy baby, and in over 95 per cent of pregnancies this is the happy result. But sometimes there is cause for anxiety, and certain diagnostic procedures can help resolve parents' fears.

I'm afraid my baby won't be normal. What procedures do I need?

Many expectant young mothers have this fear, and in most cases all that is needed is reassurance. You'll have regular antenatal check-ups at your clinic to monitor the progress of your pregnancy and resolve any doubts. However, the chances of there being an abnormality are increased if one or both parents are from families where there are instances of inherited disorders. Babies whose mothers are over 35 can also be at risk.

If my baby could be at risk, am I obliged to have any diagnostic procedures?

You will be offered any tests that are appropriate, but the decision to have them would be yours entirely; there is no obligation whatsoever. You would be counselled by your doctor, or by a genetic counsellor, who could help you assess the likelihood of there being a defect. You would very probably wish to include your partner in these discussions.

Why do birth defects occur?

A man's sperm and a woman's egg contain all the genetic (hereditary) information needed to create a new human being. This information is coded in our genes, those minuscule structures carried on the chromosomes: 23 pairs of chromosomes are inside the nucleus (the centre) of every cell in the body. One of these 23 pairs determines the sex of the fetus. If the chromosomes within this pair are in an XX configuration the baby will be a girl, XY and it will be a boy (the woman's egg always supplies an X chromosome, the sperm either another X or a Y).

Defects occur when the genes are faulty or there is an abnormal number of chromosomes. An example of a chromosomal abnormality is Down's syndrome (also known as mongolism), which occurs because the baby has 47 chromosomes instead of the usual 46. Down's syndrome is more often found in the babies of older mothers. However, some defects occur for no known reason.

How may investigations help?

Investigations help because fetal cells can be analysed to show whether or not there are any genetic or chromosomal defects.

Ultrasound* may sometimes be used, either on its own

because it can show abnormalities in the baby's body, or as a guide in conjunction with other tests. If there is a defect, then termination of pregnancy* (abortion) can be an option. If all is well, then the parents do not have to endure an anxious pregnancy, as was the case before testing when assessing the possibility of a defect was entirely a matter of weighing up the odds.

What preparations should I make for a test? I feel rather nervous about it.

Most procedures used in diagnosis are performed in the out-patient clinic of a hospital, so you can probably go home soon after. You'll only need to undress below the waist. You may be asked to have a full bladder for ultrasound to be carried out, although if the newer method using a vaginal probe (see page 14) is used this won't be necessary. You'll be fully conscious throughout whichever procedure you are having, but you won't be in any pain, and it will be over quickly. Relaxation techniques (see page 265) can help you cope with the experience. You may wish to have your partner, a relative or friend with you to give you reassurance.

Could you describe the procedures?

Ultrasound

Ultrasound is a diagnostic procedure used to monitor the development of the baby in the womb. Carried out externally, it is called a 'non-invasive' procedure, requiring no anaesthetic. (See also Chapter 1, page 13 for more about ultrasound.)

Amniocentesis

Amniocentesis is the most widely used invasive procedure. It is carried out after the fourteenth week of pregnancy; this is because the test involves withdrawing about 20 ml (2 dessert spoonfuls) of fluid from the amniotic sac which surrounds the fetus; by 14 weeks there is enough fluid to enable this much to be drawn without risk to the fetus. The amniotic fluid contains cells from the fetus, and these are then used in chromosome analysis. It takes two to four weeks to obtain the results.

HOW IT IS CARRIED OUT

First, the fetus is located by ultrasound. Then a long fine needle attached to a syringe is inserted through the abdomen and (also guided by ultrasound) into the womb (uterus). Fluid is withdrawn from the amniotic sac. A jab of local anaesthetic may be given to numb the abdomen, but usually this isn't necessary. All you'll feel is a small pricking sensation as the needle goes in; there may be a little cramping and pressure as the needle enters the womb and the fluid withdrawn from the sac. Just occasionally the needle may have to be inserted a second time, as great care is needed in locating the sac. The whole procedure takes about 15 minutes.

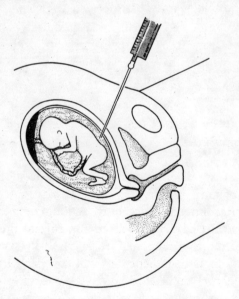

Amniocentesis involves withdrawing a sample of amniotic fluid for testing from within the amniotic sac in which the fetus floats. The procedure can be carried out after the fourteenth week of pregnancy.

Chorion Villus Sampling (CVS)

CVS is a more recent test. It can be performed as early in pregnancy as eight weeks, and the results are available much faster than with amniocentesis – sometimes within a couple of days. The parents are therefore spared an anxious wait. Early testing also means that if a pregnancy is to be terminated, the mother avoids the trauma of a late abortion. CVS takes about half an hour to carry out, and you may be given a sedative injection beforehand to help you relax.

HOW IT IS CARRIED OUT

The procedure can be performed in two ways, both guided by ultrasound.

The more usual technique is carried out through the cervix (the entrance to the womb). For this, you need to lie back with your legs comfortably apart, as for a pelvic examination*. A speculum is placed in your vagina to hold it open so the cervix can be seen. Then a narrow plastic or metal catheter (tube) is inserted into the womb via the cervix; attached to the tube is a syringe. The placenta – the organ which nourishes the fetus in the womb – is located, and a few minute fronds, called chorionic villi, are sucked from its surface. These are genetically identical to the cells of the fetus. The procedure causes only a little discomfort.

What is the other way of carrying out CVS?

This is similar to amniocentesis. A long needle attached to a syringe is inserted through the abdomen into the womb, and a sample of the chorionic villi are removed by suction. You may be given a local anaesthetic and will only feel slight pressure as the needle goes in. This technique may carry less risk of infection than the cervical method, but at the time of writing it is still being evaluated.

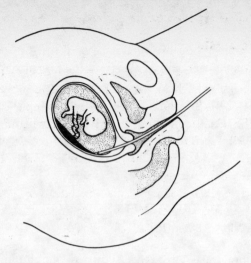

Chorion villus sampling (CVS) removes a sample of the placenta for testing. It can be performed in either of two ways: (1) via a tube inserted into the womb from the vagina, or (2) via a needle inserted through the abdomen, as for amniocentesis.

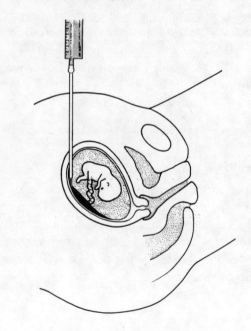

Might I be offered any other test?

Cordocentesis

Cordocentesis is a newer test which is available in specialized fetal medicine centres in some hospitals. The procedure is also called fetal blood sampling. It enables a sample of the baby's blood to be taken for testing; this is withdrawn from the umbilical cord, which contains blood vessels and connects the baby to the placenta. Cordocentesis may be carried out from about the eighteenth week of pregnancy, after which time the cord can be seen clearly by ultrasound*. You will be given a sedative first, and the procedure takes 15 to 30 minutes to carry out. The results can be obtained in just a few days.

HOW IT IS CARRIED OUT

You lie on your back and, as with amniocentesis, a long fine needle is inserted through the abdomen into the womb. A blood sample is taken from the umbilical cord. You will feel only the pricking of the needle and slight pressure.

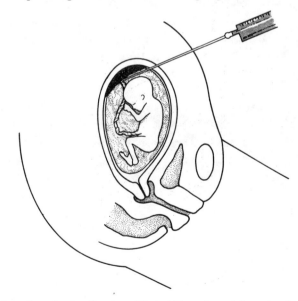

A blood sample can be taken from the umbilical cord by cordocentesis for testing after about 18 weeks of pregnancy.

Will I be all right after having one of these tests — or will it take time to recover?

Some women feel a bit shaky afterwards, which is a common emotional reaction. Others are not at all upset by the experience. If you've had a sedative you'll be drowsy, and the effects will take a few hours to wear off before you can go home. It's certainly a good idea to have someone with you who can take you home. Rest for a day if possible; you should be fully recovered after that.

I'm expecting my first baby and I belong to the Rhesus negative blood group. I've been told that I'll need an injection of a special drug after a test I'm having. Why is this?

You are one of a small number of people; most of us are Rhesus positive. Your blood group isn't a problem in itself, but if the father of your baby is Rhesus positive, rather than negative like you, your baby may be positive, too. Following any situation which could bring the baby's blood into contact with yours — for example, this test, termination*, miscarriage*, ectopic pregnancy, or childbirth (be it natural or by Caesarean* section) — you will need an injection of a drug called Anti-D within 72 hours.

The reason is that your blood and the baby's are incompatible; this is called Rhesus incompatibility. If you don't have Anti-D, your blood can form aggressive substances called antibodies against the baby's blood. These could affect not only this pregnancy, but future pregnancies as well. If you and your Rhesus-positive partner have more babies, the antibodies can attack and damage the fetal blood cells, with serious consequences. Fortunately, one jab of the drug given after any event where there could have been blood contact will stop antibodies forming, so both this and future pregnancies will be protected.

Would the drug work if my body has already built up antibodies in a previous pregnancy?

No, it would be too late. However, these tests can also be used to find out how badly affected the baby is. If necessary, the baby can be given blood transfusions in the womb by cordo-centesis; the blood is transfused via the umbilical cord. This can be a stressful procedure in itself, and so termination* could be another option. But thanks to Anti-D, Rhesus incompatibility is becoming much rarer.

Questions Women Most Often Ask About Diagnostic Procedures in Pregnancy

Are there any risks in having these tests?

All tests are carried out with the greatest care. Ultrasound* has been used worldwide for at least 20 years, with no reported effects on the mother or her unborn child. With invasive proce-dures there is inevitably the risk of a miscarriage* afterwards. With amniocentesis, the risk is put at about 1 per cent. However, with CVS or cordocentesis the risk is slightly higher, at about 2 per cent. These tests would therefore only be done when the possibility of there being a fetal defect outweighs the likelihood of losing a healthy baby. Furthermore, it is usually only women who feel they would want to terminate an abnor-mal pregnancy who would be advised to have an invasive pro-cedure. But there are exceptions: a woman expecting a much-wanted baby might wish to know in advance if s/he will be handicapped in order to make the necessary preparations for the baby's arrival and upbringing.

Which abnormalities are these tests used to detect?

As explained earlier in this chapter, ultrasound* is used on its own to examine the baby's anatomy. Modern ultrasound pic-tures are so clear that all but minor abnormalities can usually be detected. For instance, spina bifida (a spinal defect of unknown origin) is diagnosed by ultrasound. A chromosome disorder which has physical signs, such as Down's syndrome, can also be detected by ultrasound, although a further, invasive procedure would be needed to confirm this diagnosis.

Invasive procedures are most commonly used to diagnose Down's syndrome. This only affects 1 in 1000 babies born to women in their 20s, but by the time a woman is in her 40s, the risk has risen to 1 in 50. Because the risk of chromosomal abnormalities rises steeply after the age of 35, amniocentesis or CVS would normally be offered to all women over 37. A woman who has already had a Down's syndrome baby would be offered a test, regardless of her age.

There is a blood test being developed which can be carried out on a sample of the mother's blood early in the pregnancy to predict the likelihood of Down's syndrome. At the time of writing, it is not foolproof or widely available, but may be used as a pointer to whether an invasive procedure is necessary.

Cordocentesis is used to diagnose chromosome disorders, Down's syndrome again being the most common one. It is used at an advanced stage of pregnancy (over 18 weeks) when it is too late for amniocentesis or CVS.

Genetic disorders which can be detected by amniocentesis and CVS include cystic fibrosis, which affects the lungs.

These tests will show the sex of the fetus, so you will need to state clearly if you don't want to have this information. Sometimes, however, it is medically important. For example, there are hereditary disorders which only affect boys, such as haemophilia (a blood disorder) and Duchenne muscular dystrophy (which causes a progressive muscular weakness).

Certain viruses, if caught by a mother in pregnancy, can cause severe defects in the fetus, although they may produce only mild symptoms in the woman. Best known is German measles (rubella). Fetal infection can be detected by CVS.

Fortunately, you can be vaccinated against German measles before becoming pregnant, if you have not had the infection already, in which case you would be protected against it and could not be reinfected.

There seem to be an alarming number of disorders affecting the baby which can be diagnosed in pregnancy. Is it really sensible for me to become pregnant if a baby of mine could be at risk?

This is something you certainly need to discuss with your partner, doctor or a genetic counsellor before becoming pregnant. It must be stressed that even though there is a wide range of disorders which can occur, only a minority of pregnancies are affected. But you should still ensure that you are fully informed about your own situation. Some people, of course, are not deterred by the possibility of having a handicapped child. Our purpose here is simply to present the options.

Treating an Ectopic Pregnancy

What is an ectopic pregnancy?

This is where the fertilized egg implants outside the womb and starts to grow. Very occasionally it may lodge in the pelvic cavity or on an ovary or even in the cervix, but the most usual place is in one of the Fallopian tubes. This is why it is also called a tubal pregnancy. Normally fertilization takes places in one or other of the Fallopian tubes, where the sperm meets the egg. But in an ectopic pregnancy the fertilized egg then fails to move on to the womb as it should. Approximately 1 in 200 women have this type of pregnancy.

Why does it happen?

The most common reason is because the Fallopian tubes have been damaged. An infection such as pelvic inflammatory disease (PID)* can be responsible. If a sterilization* has been reversed – which means that the crushed or severed tubes have been restored by surgery – this increases the risk. Or there may be natural defects in the structure of the tubes. Should a woman conceive despite having an intra-uterine contraceptive device (IUCD) in place, which occasionally happens, there is a slightly increased risk of the pregnancy being ectopic. This may relate to the device having caused mild inflammation of the tubes. But an ectopic pregnancy is not always the result of an obvious problem.

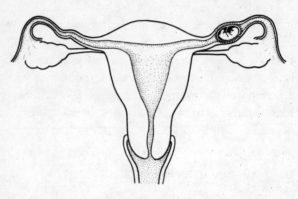

When an embryo (fertilized egg) lodges in the Fallopian tube the resulting ectopic pregnancy must be removed.

How would I know if I had an ectopic pregnancy?

The first sign is pain in the lower abdomen, often on one side. The pain may be constant or stabbing – a sign that there is bleeding from the tube; the pain becomes more severe as internal bleeding increases; there may also be spotting or bleeding from the vagina. These symptoms usually occur within the first two months, when you may not even know you are pregnant. You may have early signs of pregnancy – swollen, tender breasts, nausea and fatigue – but a routine pregnancy test may often be negative in this type of pregnancy. So, if you've had sex without contraception, or use an IUCD, and have any of these symptoms, it could be an ectopic pregnancy.

Is this a serious problem?

Yes. The tube may burst, in which case there can be serious internal bleeding. You will be in considerable pain, and might also go into shock and collapse. An ectopic pregnancy may thus be a life-threatening condition.

What should I do if I think I have an ectopic pregnancy?

See your doctor right away. If you are in very severe pain, go straight to a hospital.

How is it diagnosed?

It's not always easy to diagnose, because it can appear to be like an early miscarriage*. An ultrasound* scan may help, but more often a laparoscopy* is carried out. This allows the surgeon a direct look inside the pelvis at the tubes.

What will happen then?

The pregnancy will need to be removed. If your condition is serious, this can be an emergency operation.

Is it major surgery?

It could be called minor major surgery. If the ectopic has been diagnosed by laparoscopy* under general anaesthetic, the procedure, called a laparotomy, will follow straight on without you regaining consciousness. The surgeon makes an incision about 5 cm (2 in) across your lower abdomen just above your pubic hairline. But if the tube has not ruptured, new techniques using the laparoscope* may be carried out which avoid a laparotomy.

Could you explain the surgery for removing an ectopic pregnancy?

If the tube is still intact the ectopic may be shelled out through a small incision in the tubal wall. This may be done during a laparotomy or, as just mentioned, by new techniques using the laparoscope, which means that surgery is performed via the laparoscope without opening the abdomen for an operation. The recovery time after this surgery is therefore shorter – only about two days, i.e. no more than the length of your hospital stay. What happens is that the tube is cut open using a powerful beam of laser light, which seals as it cuts, so there is no bleeding. The pregnancy is sucked out, and the incision heals of its own accord (see illustration). If, however, the ectopic has already burst through the wall of the tube and there has been considerable bleeding, the tube will need to be removed by laparotomy. Removal of the tube is called a salpingectomy.

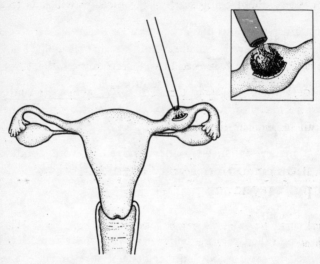

Removal of an ectopic pregnancy may be carried out by cutting open the Fallopian tube using a powerful laser beam. The embryo is then sucked out.

What sort of state will I be in after a laparotomy, and how long will I be in hospital?

This depends on how serious your condition was and how extensive the surgery. You may be in hospital for anything from four to seven days. You may need all, or none, of the following: a drain* from the incision to remove any blood remaining from a ruptured Fallopian tube; a catheter (a tube in your urethra to help you urinate); a blood transfusion* and a drip to replace fluid lost during surgery (both are given via a needle in your hand or arm).

The anaesthetic will leave you feeling groggy and perhaps rather sick, but this will pass within a day. Painkillers will be given by drip or injection, as needed, after the operation, or by mouth a day or so later. But this is not one of the more painful operations. If you were in severe pain beforehand, you'll notice the difference! You'll be up the next day, and any tubes will be removed the day after. If you're discharged a couple of days later, you will need to return to the hospital, or see your doctor, to have the stitches or clips removed from the incision. Don't worry about being scarred; the incision will fade to a fine line.

What about when I get home — do I need to convalesce?

Rest for a week, and take things easy for about a month. This means no heavy lifting (see page 111), and no driving, because this can strain your abdomen.

Questions Women Most Often Ask About Ectopic Pregnancy

I've had surgery for an ectopic pregnancy and the tube was removed. What are my chances of becoming pregnant again?

They would still be good, provided the other tube is normal, but conception may take longer because only eggs from the ovary adjacent to the remaining tube are likely to be fertilized. You can try for a pregnancy as soon as you feel able.

Can I use an IUCD contraceptive after an ectopic pregnancy?

Definitely better avoided. It's also inadvisable if you've had any form of pelvic infection. Ask your doctor or family planning clinic for advice on other contraceptive methods.

Am I likely to have an ectopic pregnancy again? I don't want to lose another baby.

It's very sad when a wanted pregnancy turns out to be ectopic. You are likely to feel cheated for a while, but your doctor or hospital can put you in touch with a counsellor or support group, if you feel you need this kind of help. Another ectopic could happen, and so your next pregnancy will need careful monitoring. An ultrasound scan* at the fifth or sixth week should show a pregnancy safe in the womb – and the odds are overwhelmingly in favour of this being the case.

If I had to have both tubes removed due to ectopic pregnancies, would this end my chances of having a baby?

You wouldn't be able to conceive in the normal way, but in vitro fertilization (IVF)* may be a possibility, as this surgical technique bypasses the Fallopian tubes. The success rate is not high and it isn't widely available, but it is worth considering if you very much want a child of your own.

Are there any medical advances which will make treating an ectopic pregnancy easier?

At the time of writing, researchers are developing a technique which ends the pregnancy without cutting open the Fallopian tube. No anaesthetic is needed and it causes only minor discomfort. A very fine flexible polythene tube is inserted via the cervix through the womb and into the affected tube. A powerful anti-cancer drug is injected down the polythene tube, directly into the ectopic. This stops it growing and it is reabsorbed by the body, leaving the Fallopian tube intact.

Caesarean Birth

When is a Caesarean birth necessary?

Only when a natural birth would be a danger to the health and life of the mother or baby. This operation removes the baby from the womb quickly and safely via an abdominal incision. Known medically as a Caesarean section, or Caesar, it may be planned in advance or carried out as an emergency operation during labour.

What are the reasons for a Caesarean?

The most usual reasons why it is carried out are:

- the baby's head is too large, or the mother's pelvis too small, to allow a vaginal birth.
- the baby is in an awkward position, e.g. breech presentation (the baby is positioned bottom or feet first), or transverse lie (the baby is lying across the womb).
- the placenta – the organ which nourishes the baby – is attached to the womb below the baby (placenta praevia) instead of above; it can cause heavy bleeding before or during labour and obstruct the birth.
- the baby is distressed during labour (short of oxygen); there is then a risk of brain damage or death to the baby. The monitor strapped to the mother's abdomen picks up a distressed fetal heartbeat.
- there is no progress in labour. Contractions may be weak, or there is one of the previous problems, or an induction of labour has failed, i.e. giving the mother hormones has not 'brought on' labour when necessary.
- the mother's health necessitates it. Heart or lung disease, or high blood-pressure, can mean that she and the baby are unfit for labour. Active herpes (an outbreak of blisters in and around the vagina) makes a natural birth unsafe because the baby can be infected.
- there are twins, triplets, or more babies; it may not be possible to deliver them vaginally.

I'm having a planned Caesarean. What preparations should I make?

This is a major operation, and you should certainly read Chapter 2 on Preparing for Surgery, bearing in mind that you will have a new baby to look after during recovery.

You will be in hospital for about 10 days, and full recovery will take a couple of months. You will tire easily for a while after the operation, and a new baby usually means broken nights too, so you will need to be able to rest during the day.

Plan to have as many domestic and family commitments taken care of as possible; have everything you need for the baby. You won't be able to do a lot of heavy shopping when you get home.

What happens in hospital before a Caesarean?

You'll be admitted the day before. Preparations are the same as for other abdominal operations, although you may be given suppositories to clear the back passage before this surgery, and your bladder also needs to be empty. A catheter* (a slim tube) is inserted into your urethra to remove urine during the operation. You will also be on a drip* throughout. You won't be given anything to eat for at least four hours before surgery, in case you vomit. Most planned Caesareans are carried out under an epidural, but occasionally circumstances call for a general anaesthetic.

What is an epidural?

It's a form of local anaesthetic which deadens all pain below the waist; it is often used in normal childbirth, and for other types of surgery. You are conscious throughout, and it can help make a Caesarean a more fulfilling experience; you will not have the after-effects of a general anaesthetic either. But not all mothers want to be awake during this major procedure. If you are worried about this, discuss it with your obstetrician (the specialist who manages your pregnancy), and read this chapter.

How is an epidural given?

It is injected into your spine at about waist level before you go into the operating theatre. You lie on your left side with your knees drawn up. A small amount of local anaesthetic is given to numb the area, then a fine hollow needle is inserted into the epidural space which surrounds the spinal cord. You will feel some pressure, but no pain, as it goes in. A fine tube is passed down the needle, then the needle is withdrawn, leaving the tube in place in the spine. Anaesthetic is injected down the tube; this will feel cold at first, and it takes effect gradually. More anaesthetic can be given via the tube as needed during surgery.

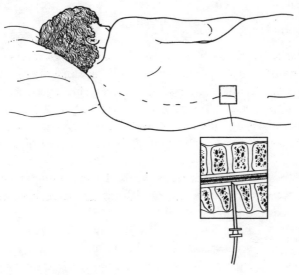

An epidural anaesthetic injected into the spine allows the mother to be fully conscious and completely pain-free during a Caesarean birth.

Sometimes a spinal anaesthetic may be used instead. This is injected deeper into the spine with a fine needle, and doesn't need 'topping up', so there is no tube. It is used less often than an epidural because it can produce unpleasant side-effects.

If I have a Caesarean under epidural, what will it be like?

In the operating theatre, your abdomen will be washed down with antiseptic and cloths arranged over it which leave only the area to be operated on exposed. A cloth screen will be placed across your midriff, so you don't have to see the operation.

There will be several people to carry out the operation and look after you. The anaesthetist and his or her assistant stand near your head; the obstetrician and his or her assistant perform the operation; there will be one or two assisting nurses and a midwife. A paediatrician (a specialist in child health) will check your baby when s/he is born. Here is what happens during the operation.

1. The anaesthetist will ensure you are properly anaesthetized by pricking your abdomen and asking if you can feel it. When the skin is completely numb, the obstetrician will clean the skin, place the sterile cloths and make the incision. The most usual place is along the top of the pubic hairline (known as a bikini incision) because it heals the best. It is about 12 cm (5 in) long, although if there is great urgency a different incision may be made, running from just below the navel to the top of the pubic hair (a midline incision).

2. When the womb is in view, the bladder is separated from it so it won't be damaged. A further incision is then made across the lower part of the womb. The amniotic sac which surrounds the fetus may already have burst, releasing fluid through your vagina, but if not it will be ruptured.

3. The obstetrician then lifts the baby's head through the incision, either with one hand or using forceps, while the assistant presses down on the top of the abdomen to help ease the baby's body out. If the baby is lying the other way round (in the breech position), the legs or bottom are lifted out first, and forceps used to cradle the head during delivery. Up to this point, the whole procedure will probably have taken no more than five minutes.

4. The umbilical cord is clamped and cut, and by this time you'll probably have seen your baby and heard his or her first cry. Sometimes it's necessary to drain mucus from the baby's nose and mouth. Breathing may not start for a minute or two, but this is not dangerous. Not all babies cry that much at birth, so don't worry if yours is quiet. If necessary, the paediatrician will help start the baby's breathing. All being well, you will be given your baby to hold.

5. Meanwhile, the afterbirth (the placenta) will have been removed and a hormone given via the drip to help your womb contract. The incision in your womb is sewn up

with soluble stitches, which dissolve away during healing. The bladder is returned to its normal position and the abdominal incision stitched or clipped. A drain* may be placed in the incision to remove liquid following the operation. All this will take about 30 to 40 minutes.

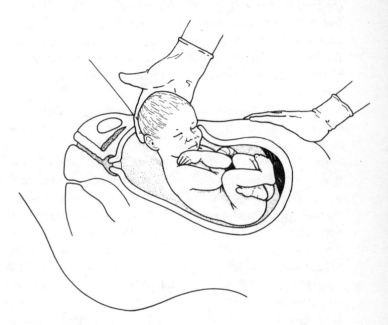

In a Caesarean birth, the obstetrician lifts the baby's head out through an incision in the lower abdomen, while an assistant presses on the abdomen to help the body to be born.

Will I feel anything at all during this operation?

With an epidural you will still be able to feel pressure and movement during the operation, but less so with a spinal because this has a deeper effect. Under an epidural you will know the moment your baby is lifted out, but there is no pain.

How will I feel afterwards, and what happens then?

Following an epidural, sensation will return gradually and you'll become aware of pain from the incision. You'll take some hours to come round from a general anaesthetic. In both situations, you'll need painkillers, which are given by drip or injection for the first day or two, and by mouth after that. You may also have needed a blood transfusion* following surgery. This is what usually happens next.

1. The drip and catheter are removed on about the second day, and the drain the day after.
2. You'll be out of bed within 24 hours, to keep your circulation going and prevent blood clots forming in your legs. The nurses will help you to start with, but soon you'll be able to manage by yourself. See page 208 for ways of easing yourself out of bed which relieve strain on your abdomen. Moving around also helps to get your digestion going again after a general anaesthetic (which tends to make it shut down). Any wind pains will (literally) pass soon. They often occur after major abdominal surgery because of air being trapped during the operation – if they are severe the nurses can provide remedies.
3. You may have cramping pains (after-pains) as your womb contracts to its pre-pregnant size. This is normal after any delivery. Breastfeeding tends to accentuate after-pains through a natural reflex, but even if you are breastfeeding you can have painkillers to reduce them.
4. You will have a blood-stained vaginal discharge for six weeks, which will steadily diminish and lighten in colour during this time. Wear maternity pads and check that there are no signs of infection, such as discolouration or a bad odour.
5. Stitches or clips will be removed between the fifth and seventh day. Your abdominal muscles will be slack, which is only to be expected. See page 211 for exercises you can do to tone them and get back your figure when you feel fit enough.
6. You and your baby will be thoroughly checked before going home.

Is it safe to breastfeed straight after a Caesarean?

Yes. Unless your baby needs special care, you can start straight away if you've had an epidural – possibly even in the operating theatre. After a general anaesthetic, the baby will be sleepy too, so feeding may take a day or two to get established. The painkillers you are taking won't damage the baby, and it's important to be comfortable if you're breastfeeding. You may be able to have your baby with you in a cot by the bed, so you'll know when s/he is hungry. If you miss a feed through tiredness, the hospital milk bank can fill the gap.

How careful do I have to be when I get home?

You do need to take things easy for about a month and not lift anything heavy for at least six weeks (see pages 111–12). If someone can stay with you and help look after the baby and the home, this will be a great advantage. If not, you will need a home help; ask your doctor or the hospital social worker about this if necessary. Hopefully, you will also be able to rely on your partner, family and friends. But you probably won't want many visitors right away, so say you'll let them know how you and the baby are doing and if you need any help.

Questions Women Most Often Ask About Caesarean Birth

Can my partner be present at the delivery?

It's usually permitted if you're having an epidural, but he needs to be aware that this is a major procedure. It depends on your obstetrician; having another person in the operating theatre is not always an advantage.

I am very disappointed that I had to have a Caesarean. I wanted a natural birth and feel I've failed somehow. It's also made me less fond of my new baby.

These feelings are not uncommon, but you are not a failure. Your baby had to be born this way and it wasn't your fault. If s/he needed special care, or you had a general anaesthetic and could not hold him or her at birth, you may not have maternal feelings right away. In any event, it's not unusual to feel a bit depressed after childbirth before your hormones return to normal. There may be a Caesarean support group in your area (or you could start one); talking to other Caesarean mothers may help you see this in a positive light. But if these feelings persist, tell your doctor, as help can be given.

Will a natural delivery be possible next time?

The majority of reasons for carrying out a Caesarean do not recur, and so a natural birth may well be possible. It also depends on how many Caesareans you have had; there can be a danger of the scar in the womb giving way during labour. You may be able to have what's called 'a trial of labour' and, if it goes well, a natural delivery. You will need to give birth in hospital in case there are complications and another Caesarean is required. But it has to be said that because there is increasing litigation against doctors as a result of birth injuries to babies delivered naturally, there is more pressure on doctors to perform Caesareans – particularly as they are becoming safer for the mother too. Often, the parents themselves will request a Caesarean – for example, if there is a breech presentation.

How many Caesareans is it safe to have?

The risk of complications increases slightly with each Caesarean. Sterilization* may be recommended after three such deliveries, but your obstetrician will advise you.

Will I be left very scarred if I have more than one Caesarean?

No. The incision is usually made in the same place and the old scar tissue cut away. The new scar will also fade.

I'm worried about restarting sex because I don't feel like it at all after my Caesarean.

This is hardly surprising. Give yourself about four to six weeks. You need time to heal inside and regain your energy. It is still important to be physically close and affectionate to your partner during this time. He will be adjusting to the changes a new baby brings and coping while you are less active. He should not be made to feel emotionally excluded because you are preoccupied with the baby and recovery.

When you first try intercourse, a lubricant will help, because your vagina may be dry until hormone levels adjust after childbirth. Find comfortable positions which don't put pressure on your incision; try lying side by side, or with your back to him. Penetration need not be so deep in these positions, and if you still feel a bit tender inside, there will be less pushing on the womb. You need to use contraception right away, as you can become pregnant, even before your periods start again.

Do seek help from your doctor if negative feelings or any physical discomfort continue.

I've had a Caesarean and would like more children. How soon can I become pregnant?

It's advisable to wait about a year to allow the womb to heal fully.

Was Julius Caesar the first Caesarean birth?

Probably not, because in Roman times the operation was only performed to deliver the child from a dead mother; there is good evidence that Caesar's mother Aurelia was still alive when he invaded Britain in 55 BC. There are many (and conflicting) theories about the origin of the word, but it may have come from the Latin 'caedare', meaning 'to cut'. Of course, many famous people have been born this way!

Episiotomy

Could you explain what this is?

An episiotomy is a surgical procedure which may be needed during normal childbirth to ease delivery of the baby. It is an incision made from the lower edge of the vagina into the perineum (the area between the vagina and the anus).

When is an episiotomy necessary?

In the last stages of labour the baby's head enters the vagina, which must stretch to its full extent so the baby can be born. At this point an episiotomy may be necessary for the following reasons.

- The vagina may tear. Small, superficial tears are not generally a problem and usually heal well. If a deeper tear looks like being severe enough to extend into the back passage, the incision is made to prevent damage to the anal muscles.
- The baby needs to be delivered by forceps. This instrument is used to grip the head on either side so the obstetrician can help deliver the baby. An episiotomy allows room for the forceps.
- The baby is distressed due to lack of oxygen; the incision widens the vaginal exit and hastens the birth.
- The baby is premature and has a softer head; an episiotomy reduces vaginal pressure on the baby's skull.

How is an episiotomy carried out, and will it be painful?

The incision is carried out using obstetrical scissors. It's no more than 3 cm (1½ in) long, and is made on either the midline (a straight line between the vagina and anus) or mediolaterally (to one side of the anus). Local anaesthetic is given first, so it won't hurt at all; further anaesthetic is not needed if you've had an epidural*.

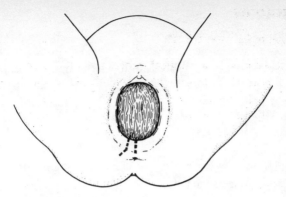

To ease delivery of the baby's head, an episiotomy incision may be made either on a straight line (the midline) between the vagina and anus, or to one side (mediolaterally).

What happens to the cut after my baby is born?

The area is thoroughly cleansed and examined; more anaesthetic is given if necessary. The cut is then stitched together in layers, using soluble stitches which are absorbed during healing.

I've heard that an episiotomy can hurt a lot afterwards. How long does this go on for, and can it be relieved?

It shouldn't be too painful, although it will be sore. Taking a painkiller such as paracetamol will help. The cut will heal within a few days. Here are some ways to relieve discomfort and promote healing.

- Keep the area clean. Wash gently and thoroughly (a hand-held shower head or bidet is best for this) after defecation; use unscented, non-irritating soap. Dry yourself using a blow dryer set on its coolest setting, this avoids the need to touch the area with a cloth or towel.
- Change your maternity pads frequently.
- Salt in your bath will be beneficial and soothing; use two heaped tablespoons in shallow water, about 7.5 cm (3 in) deep.
- Apply a soothing vitamin E cream.

- Ice packs will help relieve soreness.
- Eat a sensible, high-fibre diet to avoid constipation, because straining will hurt; use suppositories if necessary.
- Sit on a rubber-ring cushion for the first few days.

Questions Women Most Often Ask About Episiotomy

Will my vagina be weakened by the cut? Could it tear again during intercourse? These worries are a real turn-off.

Physical discomfort in this area is bound to influence sexual response, but you should feel able to try gentle intercourse in about six weeks. A lubricant will help relieve any discomfort; the vagina is dryer at this time anyway, due to altered hormonal levels. If there is any pain, tell your doctor. The cut won't weaken your vagina, and there's no danger of intercourse causing it to tear again.

I had an episiotomy with my first baby. Will I need it again?

If any of the reasons given earlier recur, it may be needed again, but it is much less likely with a second baby because the vagina usually stretches more easily and tears less.

Do many women have to have an episiotomy? I'd prefer not to if possible.

No, many women give birth without one. It used to be carried out almost routinely because it was thought to prevent prolapse and pelvic relaxation* occurring in later life. It's now known that these problems result from damage higher up in the birth canal. If you are worried about having an episiotomy, discuss it first with your obstetrician or midwife, so that they know how you feel and can respect your wishes as far as possible.

6

PROLAPSE AND PELVIC RELAXATION

Prolapse and pelvic relaxation describe what can happen if the pelvic floor muscles become slack (relaxed) and/or the ligaments and muscles holding the womb in place are weakened. The word prolapse means fall, and the pelvic organs – the womb, vagina, bladder, urethra and bowel – can sag and bulge out of place, although it is most likely to affect the womb, which can slip down into the vagina (a uterine prolapse), sometimes pulling down the other organs with it. This causes discomfort and unpleasant symptoms which interfere with normal life.

Many women experience mild symptoms of prolapse and pelvic relaxation. Fortunately, really severe problems occur much less often nowadays. Self-help methods can do much to prevent these problems, or relieve mild symptoms, and we give them here. But repair surgery is sometimes recommended, and is well worth having if you are experiencing debilitating symptoms.

What causes prolapse and pelvic relaxation?

Pregnancy and childbirth place stress on the pelvic muscles and ligaments, which also soften at this time as a result of hormones. In addition to their usual job of holding the pelvic organs in place, they carry the weight of the fetus, and are pushed, stretched and may be torn during labour. Sometimes they do not return to normal afterwards if they have been over-stretched or torn.

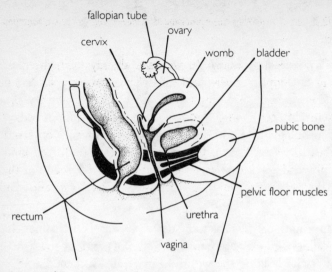

Normal position of the pelvic organs and supporting muscles.

If pregnancy and childbirth are thought to be the main causes, why do middle-aged women tend to have these problems?

A uterine prolapse tends to happen in middle age because the muscles and ligaments holding the womb in place can weaken then anyway. The hormone oestrogen, secreted by the ovaries, helps keep them supple and strong, but levels of this hormone drop during and after the menopause, so any damage done earlier is likely to become more obvious. Hormone replacement therapy (HRT)*, where the woman is given substitute ovarian hormones, may help prevent this problem in some women.

Do these problems ever affect women who have not had children?

Women without children can occasionally develop a prolapse, possibly due to the hormonal changes of the menopause, or an inherited tendency, or simply the pull of gravity. Sometimes the same physical stresses which cause hernias in men can damage the pelvic muscles in women. Very strenuous sports or heavy lifting may do this, but these problems are more likely to occur in women who have had children.

How likely am I to develop these problems if I have children? It's a worrying thought.

There's no need to worry. As we have already said, the chances of your developing severe problems of this kind are far less now than they used to be. This is because of better delivery procedures in childbirth. Also, women have fewer children today, so these problems do not occur simply as a result of repeated childbearing. And fortunately women no longer do the kind of hard physical work that was once quite usual for many of them, and which strained pelvic floor muscles before and after childbirth.

I am pregnant and want to know what I can do to strengthen my pelvic muscles.

There are exercises which strengthen your pelvic floor muscles. These exercises can benefit all women, and are described later in this chapter (see pages 112–14). You can also learn them at antenatal classes given by your hospital or as recommended by your doctor. You will also be taught special breathing and relaxation techniques which will make labour much easier and help prevent damage to your pelvic floor.

I've heard that having an episiotomy* during labour can prevent prolapse and pelvic relaxation. Is this true?

It was once thought to help, but this is no longer so. Making a surgical cut into the perineum (the area between the vagina and the rectum) to allow the baby's head to emerge more easily does not prevent damage to the muscles higher up in the birth canal, which are the ones mainly affected by these problems.

I have an embarrassing problem following my baby's birth. I find that when I cough, sneeze or laugh suddenly, or do anything strenuous, I wet myself slightly. Why is this happening?

This is called stress incontinence, and is often associated with

mild prolapse and pelvic relaxation. Even though you are probably very busy with a new baby, you should find time to do the
strengthening exercises given later in this chapter (page 112),
and which you will probably have been taught at ante- and
postnatal classes. These exercises are very important in restoring
pelvic muscle tone after childbirth, and are often all that is necessary to relieve this problem. But you should also see your
doctor, for two reasons. First, to ensure that this really is the
cause of the problem and, second, so that s/he can check on the
degree of your prolapse and pelvic relaxation. This will mean
having a pelvic examination*, which will enable the doctor to
see the problem very quickly.

I was told after a routine pelvic examination that I have a mildly prolapsed
womb. I wasn't aware of this. Will anything need to be done?*

It's not uncommon to have a mild prolapse, and it doesn't necessarily cause any symptoms. If it isn't bothering you, then
nothing needs to be done, but your doctor will want to keep a
check on it, and you should report any symptoms that occur.
You should also ensure that you adopt a healthier lifestyle, if
you need to, because this can help prevent a prolapse from getting worse.

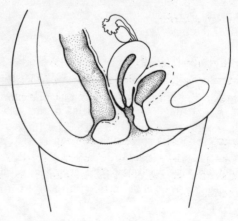

A mildly prolapsed womb descends into the top of the vagina.

Why does adopting a healthier lifestyle help prevent prolapse from getting worse? How can this have any direct effect on my womb?

It can have a very direct effect because factors such as a poor diet, being overweight and smoking can all lead to increased pressure on the muscles and ligaments holding the womb in place, which can in turn aggravate any existing problems. A diet lacking in fibre (roughage) can result in constipation, and repeated straining will cause the womb to 'bear down'. If you are overweight, this also increases pressure inside the abdomen. And, in addition to all its other damaging effects, smoking makes you cough, and persistent coughing will put pressure on the pelvic muscles. Advice on healthier living is given in Chapter 18.

I feel very tired and have a dragging sensation in my pelvis. I also get backache if I stand for long. Is my prolapsed womb causing these problems, and are there any ways I can help myself?

Yes it is and, yes, there are some ways of helping yourself. Good posture and wearing a girdle can help. Rest with your feet up whenever possible. Yoga exercises, such as head and shoulder stands, can relieve discomfort, but not everyone can do them. Kneeling forwards with your hips raised higher than your head may also help. But these are not long-term solutions: you should see your doctor.

It's becoming very difficult for me and my partner to have sex because of my prolapse. Full penetration is impossible, and his penis pushing on my womb is most uncomfortable. My vagina is loose and we both have difficulty reaching orgasm.

See your doctor. These problems can be put right and you need to discuss the options with your doctor. Also read the question-and-answer section at the end of this chapter, which deals with problems such as this.

You say that surgery is sometimes recommended. When is this likely to be necessary?

When symptoms have reached the stage where other methods are not beneficial and the woman is experiencing problems that make life increasingly difficult. The previous two questions cover some of the major problems which require surgery. Here is a description of other serious difficulties that can occur. If the bladder and urethra – the passage thorough which you urinate – have prolapsed into the front wall of the vagina (a cysto-urethrocele), stress incontinence may be a problem. Emptying the bladder can also be difficult unless the woman inserts a finger into her vagina to support the bulge when urinating. Urinary infections, which cause cystitis (pain on urination), can thus become more likely.

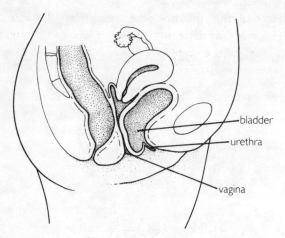

Prolapse of the bladder and urethra into the front vaginal wall (a cysto-urethrocele).

Similarly, if the muscular wall of the vagina supporting the rectum is weakened, the bowel can bulge into the back of the vagina (a rectocele). Defecation will be very uncomfortable and, again, the woman may need to support the bulge with her finger to make it possible, although incontinence is not a problem with a rectocele.

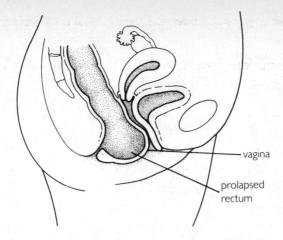

Prolapse of the bowel (rectum) into the back vaginal wall (a rectocele) makes defecation very uncomfortable.

In a severe uterine prolapse, the womb can descend so low in the vagina that any straining pushes it out of the entrance. The woman may need to replace it in her vagina and may feel as if she is 'losing her insides'.

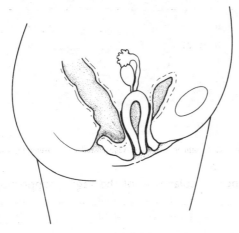

In a severe uterine prolapse, the womb can be so low in the vagina that the cervix appears at the entrance.

All these problems can be corrected by repair surgery, but a woman would be well advised to seek medical help before they become this serious.

However, discomfort is not necessarily related to the severity of the problems. Some women with milder prolapse and pelvic relaxation can actually have more discomfort. In such cases, repair surgery can be just as helpful and necessary.

Does repair surgery leave any scars?

Repair surgery for prolapse is done via the vagina, so there is no visible scarring. Surgery for stress incontinence can be carried out through the abdomen via an incision along the pubic hairline. This leaves a thin scar which will be hidden by underwear or a bikini (thus called a bikini scar). It fades with time anyway.

I've been told I need repair surgery and am very worried. What will happen, and how long will I be in hospital?

The type of operation depends on your particular problem, but repair surgery is always done under general anaesthetic and you will be in hospital for about a week, so do read Chapter 2 on Preparing for Surgery. The next four questions will inform and reassure you about the operations.

I have a prolapse of the bladder and urethra and am having surgery. How is this carried out, and will it be painful?

You have a cysto-urethrocele. This can be repaired by a straightforward operation called anterior repair (or anterior colporraphy). This involves simply removing the sagging vaginal skin and tissue, usually formed in a diamond shape. The underlying supportive tissue and the skin edges are then brought together and stitched with soluble stitches, which dissolve away during healing. This 'tightening-up' operation pushes and lifts the bladder and urethra back into position.

It can be described as intermediate-to-major surgery, but you should not have any severe pain or discomfort. You may need a catheter (a tube inserted in the urethra to help you urinate) for a day or two. You may also be on a drip* immediately after surgery, to replace fluid lost during the operation. As with most operations, you will be encouraged to get out of bed and walk around within a couple of days of surgery.

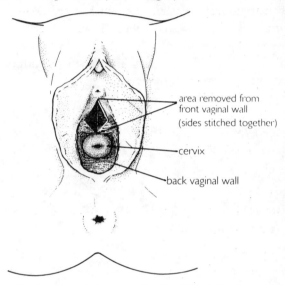

area removed from front vaginal wall (sides stitched together)

cervix

back vaginal wall

To repair a cysto-urethrocele, a diamond-shaped area of sagging skin and tissue is removed from inside the front vaginal wall, and the edges and underlying tissue are stitched together; this lifts the bladder and urethra back into place.

Even though I don't have a severe prolapse of the bladder and urethra, I have a problem with stress incontinence which I'm told needs surgery. What sort of operation will be done?

There does not necessarily have to be a severe cysto-urethrocele for there to be a problem with stress incontinence. Even so, the purpose of surgery is to lift up the tissue around the base of the bladder where the urethra starts; this is called the neck of the bladder.

The surgeon's technique and experience will influence his or her choice of operation. Some surgeons will want to do this operation through the vagina – a modified form of anterior colporraphy known as a Pacey repair. This involves buttressing the bladder by bringing tissue together from the sides of the vagina and stitching it with soluble stitches. This lifts the neck of the bladder.

Alternatively, a surgeon may wish to operate via the abdomen, which leaves a bikini scar. In this operation (called colposuspension), permanent stitches are placed each side of the vagina and then attached to the ligaments at each side of the pubic bone; these stitches lift the vagina and the neck of the bladder with it. This operation is being performed more often because it is more effective.

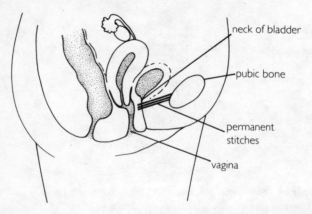

neck of bladder

pubic bone

permanent stitches

vagina

Stress incontinence (leakage) due to a mild cysto-urethrocele can be treated by an abdominal operation called colposuspension. Permanent stitches placed either side of the vagina are attached to the ligaments each side of the pubic bone, lifting the neck of the bladder.

Whichever operation you have, you will need a catheter afterwards to help you urinate. This may be inserted into the urethra, although some surgeons will place it in the bladder through the abdomen. The latter method allows the woman to try to urinate normally while the catheter is in place (the bladder heals naturally once it is removed). Women often worry if they are not able to pass urine right away, but this is quite usual and not a cause for concern. You will have a catheter for about five days while you are in hospital.

I am having a rectocele repaired and want to know what this involves.

This operation is similar to the anterior repair, but is carried out on the back wall of the vagina, and so is called a posterior repair (posterior colpoperineorraphy, but don't worry about pronouncing it). A triangle of sagging skin and tissue is taken away from inside the vagina, down to and including its junction with the perineum. The edges are then stitched together, along with the muscles of the perineum underneath, using soluble stitches. This restores the bowel to its normal position.

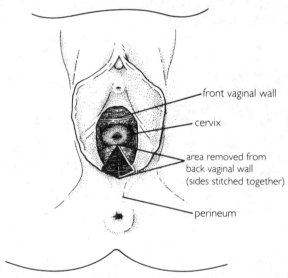

A rectocele repair involves removing a triangle of sagging skin and tissue from inside the back vaginal wall, down to the perineum. The skin edges, along with the muscles of the perineum, are stitched together, thus restoring the bowel to its normal position.

There is more discomfort after this operation – it's rather like having stitches after childbirth; you feel sore and a bit raw. You may need to insert suppositories into the rectum during healing to help defecation, as any straining would be painful and could disrupt the repair. Applying ice-packs to the perineum can relieve discomfort, and using vitamin E cream is thought by some to help healing. A rubber ring cushion can make sitting easier.

Although this operation may sound off-putting, any short-term discomfort is worth the long-term result: you will be free of the awkward and unpleasant symptoms which were caused by the rectocele.

What will be done to repair my prolapsed womb? I hear it's a big operation, and I'm dreading it.

Don't dread it, because you will feel so much better for having had it done. The type of operation depends on several factors. If the womb is not low in the vagina, or if the woman wants to retain her womb, or if she's frail and perhaps elderly, a Fothergill (or Manchester) repair may be carried out. This is one and the same operation: Fothergill is the name of the surgeon who devised it, Manchester the place where he worked.

The operation is done via the vagina. The womb is detached from the ligaments which support it at the sides, and the cervix (the neck of the womb) is then removed, which makes the womb shorter. A tuck is taken in the supporting ligaments to shorten them, and they are reattached to the womb, using soluble stitches. This raises the womb in the vagina and pulls up sagging skin. The vagina is then packed with a gauze dressing and a catheter is inserted in the urethra to help urination.

You probably won't feel too special afterwards – that is, until the gauze dressing and catheter have been removed, usually within 48 hours. You may also be on a drip*. You will of course be encouraged to get out of bed and walk around soon after the operation. You will spend seven to ten days in hospital and will probably feel much more comfortable by the end of the week.

Would I still be able to have children after a Fothergill/Manchester repair?

It's still possible, although the risks of a miscarriage* would be increased as the cervix has been removed. Childbirth would very likely be by Caesarean section* (the baby is delivered via an incision in the abdomen), because a natural birth could cause the problems to recur. However, by the time repair surgery is necessary, a woman is usually at an age when she has completed her family.

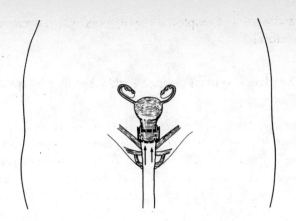

(1) The Fothergill/Manchester repair raises the womb in the vagina.

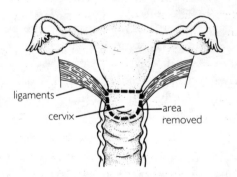

(2) Before. The womb is detached from its slack supporting ligaments and the cervix is removed.

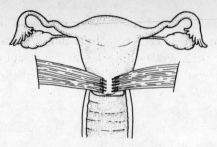

(3) After. The ligaments have been shortened and re-attached to the womb, holding it in position

How is a severe prolapse of the womb treated?

Where the womb is very low in the vagina, and when there may be other reasons for removing it, a vaginal hysterectomy is the best treatment because it is more likely to be a permanent cure than a Fothergill/Manchester repair.

In a vaginal hysterectomy, the womb is removed via the vagina; this is major surgery. Removing the womb can also have a deep emotional impact on some women, and so you do need to be fully prepared both physically and emotionally if you are having a hysterectomy. Read Chapter 15 on Hysterectomy, which gives detailed advice and information on coping positively with this operation.

You have described several operations which correct prolapse and pelvic relaxation. Are they ever carried out all at once?

Yes, but of course it depends on the extent of the problems. A Fothergill/Manchester repair, or a hysterectomy, may be combined with other repair operations as necessary. This does make for more discomfort initially, but it also resolves all the problems at the same time.

Are there likely to be any complications following a repair?

The vagina is not a sterile environment, so it is possible for infection to occur. Heavy bleeding about ten days after surgery for a prolapsed womb is a sign of this. Try not to be frightened if this happens – it can be dealt with quickly. Call your doctor right away; you may need to go back into hospital for a day or two. A gauze pack will be inserted in your vagina to stop the bleeding, and you'll be given antibiotics. Sometimes antibiotics are given routinely to guard against this problem. A certain amount of blood-stained discharge is normal, however, and may go on for several weeks. You need to wear sanitary towels, not tampons, to help prevent infection.

Another problem which may occur after repair surgery for prolapse or stress incontinence is a urinary infection, which can result in pain or a burning sensation when you urinate (cystitis). Operating on this area can cause bruising, which makes it susceptible to infection. Any urinary problems should be reported to your doctor straight away, and will also be treated with antibiotics.

Questions Women Most Often Ask About Prolapse and Pelvic Relaxation

Is there anything I can do to help myself recover from prolapse repair surgery?

It's a question of not doing, rather than doing. Avoid any heavy lifting for six months, as this will damage the repair work. This means not lifting anything which uses your abdominal and pelvic floor muscles. You'll be very much aware of any strain on these muscles straight after surgery because they will hurt if you attempt more than they're ready to handle. But you'll become less sensitive as you heal, and this is when you need to be careful. Here are some practical guidelines.

- Don't carry any heavy household shopping. When shopping in a supermarket, always use a trolley, not a handbasket. In some supermarkets an assistant may be available to reload your trolley at the checkout, wheel it to your car and help you unload it into the car. If you shop without a car, or prefer traditional shops and stores to supermarkets, invest in a trolley bag (a shopping bag on wheels); there are some attractive designs now, so it doesn't have to look geriatric.

- Housework can be a problem, so it could be worth having a home help to tide you over. In any event, don't attempt to move any furniture, turn mattresses, or lift your vacuum cleaner round corners – push it along the floor and get someone to take it upstairs (if necessary) for you.
- If you like gardening, confine yourself to pruning and light weeding; don't do any digging, mowing or hedge-cutting.
- If you are in a job, don't go back to work until your doctor advises, and even then – if you work in an office – don't carry a heavy briefcase or files for six months; if you work in a shop or factory, don't lift anything heavy off the floor or from a high shelf.

When you have recovered, always lift heavy objects correctly; it will spare your back as well as your pelvic floor muscles.

What is the correct way to lift something heavy?

Get as close to it as possible. Bend at the knees into a squatting position, keeping your back straight – or you can go down on one knee if this is easier. Lift the object, holding it close to you, using the muscles of your arms and shoulders (not your back) – using your leg muscles to stand up. Above all, don't bend from the waist and haul the object off the floor – this will cause strains. And certainly don't lift anything which is so heavy that it really is a struggle.

Could you describe the exercises which can strengthen pelvic floor muscles before and after childbirth?

These are simple exercises which can be both a test and a treatment. Note that the muscles of the buttocks, thighs and abdomen are not involved in any of these exercises, so make sure you are exercising the muscles which surround the vagina, urethra and rectum.

1. When urinating, try doing it in short, sharp bursts by alternately contracting your pelvic floor muscles to stop the flow of urine and then releasing them. If you can't do this, your pelvic floor muscles definitely need strengthening and you should practise this exercise as often as possible.

2. If you can do the first exercise, try interrupting the flow of urine and holding it to a count of five before 'letting go'. The more you do this exercise, the more you will strengthen your pelvic floor muscles.

3. You can also exercise these muscles against a resistant object. This involves inserting an object, such as a tampon applicator, part way into your vagina and holding it there. Then you do exactly the same exercise as when urinating: you clench and relax the muscles that would interrupt urination, only this time your aim is to grip the resistant object.

How many times should I do these exercises?

These exercises were devised some years ago by Dr Arnold Kegel, an American gynaecologist, and so are often called Kegel exercises. He recommended doing 300 a day to prevent stress incontinence, and invented a special resistant object called a perineometer, which recorded the strength of contractions. There are modern versions of this device which give highly accurate readings. But whether or not you try one of these, or simply use a tampon applicator (or a vibrator, if you prefer), you'll soon find you can do the exercises without a resistant object. This means you can practise wherever you are, whatever you're doing, and no one will know. Keeping count is not easy, but don't worry too much about this, so long as you can do all the exercises described here.

Can these exercises help if you've had repair surgery for prolapse and pelvic relaxation?

Yes, they can. They will strengthen the muscles after surgery and help prevent problems recurring. You should start them as soon as you feel able to.

How can these exercises benefit all women, as you said earlier?

Originally, when humans walked on all fours, these muscles did not have to support the pelvic organs to anything like the same extent. They have never completely adapted to this role in a standing position, which is why strengthening them can benefit all women, even those who have no children.

A significant bonus, which is given more emphasis in sex manuals than in books on women's health, is that strong pelvic floor muscles can enhance your sexual pleasure. Gynaecological problems and surgery can have a very negative effect on sexual desire, and so can the experience of childbirth sometimes. These exercises therefore have the added value of increasing your sexual sensitivity, making it easier for you to respond and have orgasms.

Can sex ever cause prolapse and pelvic relaxation, or make them worse?

No, never − however vigorous it is.

I'm having a prolapse repair and I want it to improve my sex life. But before my aunt had her operation some years ago, she told the doctor that she had no wish to be 'sexually active'. Does this make any difference to the operation?

This is something which your gynaecologist will certainly discuss with you. Repair surgery tightens the vagina, and in a woman who does not wish to be sexually active, the repair can be made tighter still.

You wish to continue your sex life, and an efficient repair can be done which allows for intercourse. The problems which spoiled lovemaking will be resolved, and you and your partner will again be able to enjoy sex.

Repair surgery is most often needed by women who are past the menopause, but few doctors today would simply accept without question that it is 'normal' for an older woman, such as your aunt, not to want sex. A woman who thinks she has finished with it must be absolutely sure about this. It may be that the physical discomfort caused by prolapse and pelvic relaxation has put her off. Vaginal dryness due to the hormonal changes of the menopause can make any discomfort worse, but this can also be resolved. Or it may be that sexual and emotional problems with her partner are turning her off; these could be treated by sex therapy and counselling. Or she might be without a partner and so have lost interest through lack of opportunity.

The options must be carefully considered, and if a woman is in any doubt, allowance will be made for the possibility that she might want to change her mind later.

When is it all right to have intercourse after repair surgery? My partner wants to restart sex, but I'm worried that it will hurt.

You'll have a follow-up appointment about six weeks after surgery and will probably be given the all-clear then. But this doesn't mean that lovemaking has to cease before this. There are of course other ways of making love without penetration. Physical and emotional closeness is often especially important during times of stress, such as after surgery.

When you restart intercourse, your partner will need to be gentle at first. If you are tense because of your fears, you are likely to feel discomfort. Try to relax. Using a lubricant, such as KY jelly, will ease any discomfort, but sex shouldn't hurt. Doing the pelvic floor exercises will tell you when your pelvic muscles have ceased to be uncomfortable. As these are the muscles which repeatedly contract during orgasm, you may feel the contractions more sharply to start with, but you shouldn't be in any pain. In fact, the long-term results of surgery will be a much-improved sex life.

Is it always possible to operate for prolapse and pelvic relaxation?

Not always. It may be inadvisable to operate, perhaps because a general anaesthetic could be risky for a woman who is elderly or frail. Sometimes, however, a way round this can be found by giving an epidural* instead; this is a local anaesthetic injected into the spine which numbs the body from the waist down so that surgery can be carried out with the woman fully conscious.

But if the stress of surgery would be too great, then a ring pessary made of firm rubber or plastic is inserted high in the vagina. It is like a diaphragm contraceptive, but without the dome. This supports the sagging pelvic organs. If it causes any irritation, a cream containing the hormone oestrogen may help, if its use is carefully controlled. A ring pessary can also be used by women who do not want to have surgery. It needs to be removed and cleaned about every three months, either by the woman herself or at a clinic.

If you've ever had a hysterectomy to remove the womb, could you ever have prolapse problems afterwards — or would this be impossible without a womb?

It is most unlikely but not impossible. Very occasionally the vaginal walls may sag when the womb has been removed, but this would usually happen only years later, maybe not until after the menopause. Surgery to correct this problem would most likely be carried out through the vagina, as for anterior and/or posterior repair (see page 104 and page 107). Some surgeons may choose to operate through the abdomen to relieve the problem by securing the top of the vagina to the pelvic bone. Recovery from this operation would be the same as for hysterectomy; see Chapter 15.

7

TERMINATION OF PREGNANCY

When an unwanted pregnancy is ended by medical means, it is called an induced abortion or termination of pregnancy. Our aim here is to explain how it is carried out and to give reassurance about the procedures involved. Abortion is still a controversial subject even in countries where it has been legalized, while in some countries it remains illegal. The purpose of this chapter is not to debate the moral arguments for and against abortion, nor to explore the reasons why a pregnancy may be unwanted. A woman who is in this situation and in a country where there is safe, legal abortion is entitled to the help of expert counselling and medical advice.

What should I do first if I think I have an unwanted pregnancy?

If you have early signs of pregnancy – a missed period, swollen, tender breasts and, sometimes, nausea, frequency of urination and fatigue – the first thing you need to do is find out for sure whether you are pregnant. You must not delay, because if there is an unwanted pregnancy you need to find out as soon as possible.

Where should I seek help?

Your own doctor can do a pregnancy test, and is often the most helpful and reassuring person in this situation. But if you have reservations about seeing him or her you can go to a family planning clinic or pregnancy advisory service. Whoever you see will treat this as an absolutely confidential matter.

Some pharmacists do pregnancy testing, or you can buy a home testing kit, but either way you will not have the support and guidance of an experienced person to help you cope if the result is positive. Also, a home kit may not be as accurate as a test carried out by professionals.

How is a pregnancy test done?

Simply collect a sample of urine in a clean, dry container. The first morning specimen is best, as it is likely to be the most concentrated in hormones. The test measures a hormone called human chorionic gonadotrophin (HCG), which is present only during pregnancy. An accurate result can be obtained by testing from the day your period was due, or possibly even a few days prior to your expected period.

If an unwanted pregnancy is confirmed, what is the next step?

Again, you should discuss the result with your doctor, family planning clinic or a pregnancy advisory service. You may be referred to a gynaecologist. Counselling will be provided and you must be prepared to talk openly about your situation and feelings. The practical aspects of a termination will be explained; these include the legal requirements which have to be met before a termination can be carried out, and any fees payable for the operation – although free abortion may be available; ask about this if necessary.

Can I expect to be treated sympathetically?

Yes. Many women are glad of the opportunity to talk things over in confidence with a sympathetic doctor or counsellor, and have their questions answered. If, however, you feel you are not being treated sympathetically, or you are not happy about the information and advice you are given, you can see another doctor, or go to a different clinic or advisory service.

You may also want to talk things over with a partner or others who are close to you. Their support can be most valuable. But the decision to terminate a pregnancy is rarely an easy one, and many women find they have conflicting emotions, so don't involve people who may just add to your stress.

What legal requirements must be met?

These depend on the country in which you live. The doctors involved in assessing the reasons for a termination must be convinced that your case meets these requirements. If you are not satisfied with their assessment, you can ask for a second opinion. Of course, you also have the right to say what you think, just as everyone has the right to campaign for changes to the law if they consider it necessary.

In Britain, for instance, the law requires that the following risks in continuing the pregnancy must be greater than the risk in terminating it: the risk to your life or to your physical or mental health, or to that of any child(ren) you may already have. If there is a substantial risk that the child will be born with a severe physical or mental handicap, this is also grounds for a termination.

Are there any other preliminaries before a termination?

It's essential for your own safety that the doctor and gynaecologist have your full medical history, if this is not already known, and you will be asked a wide range of questions about your health and any previous pregnancies. Routine health checks will also be carried out. Some of these can be done at the hospital or clinic where you will be having the abortion, so you may need to make a visit there before the operation.

You will be given a pelvic examination*. Tests for infection will be made because, if undetected, an infection could enter your reproductive tract during the operation. You may need another pregnancy test to ensure you really are pregnant. Your blood-pressure will be taken, and tests will be done on your blood and urine.

How is a termination carried out?

The length of time you have been pregnant will determine which procedure is used. The earlier a termination can be carried out, the safer it is, which is why it is so important not to delay seeking help. The doctor can often tell how advanced a pregnancy is by feeling the womb (uterus), although the usual way a pregnancy can be dated is by counting from the first day of the last normal period.

Could you describe the procedures used in an early termination?

Vacuum Suction

Vacuum suction (also called vacuum aspiration or suction curettage) can be used up to 12 weeks; this is called the first trimester (three months) of pregnancy.

The procedure can be carried out on a day-patient basis under a local anaesthetic, or under general anaesthetic, in which case you may stay in overnight. The type of anaesthetic to be used can be discussed with your gynaecologist; some women are worried about being conscious, and so a general anaesthetic will be better for them. Doctors also have their preferences, but the woman's feelings should be taken into account. Even if a local anaesthetic is planned, you will still be asked not to eat anything for about four hours before the operation. This is in case a general anaesthetic is necessary, as fasting prevents you vomiting when under anaesthetic. See Chapter 2 on Preparing for Surgery.

How is a vacuum suction termination performed?

You will be asked to undress and put on a surgical gown, but it isn't necessary to shave your pubic hair. The whole operation lasts no more than 15 to 20 minutes, and the actual abortion procedure takes only about five minutes.

If a local anaesthetic is to be used, a sedative may be injected into your buttock or thigh beforehand to help you relax. When a termination can be done within seven weeks of the start of the pregnancy it is a very straightforward procedure, and a local anaesthetic is often used.

You lie on your back with your legs supported apart by stirrups. The vaginal area is wiped with a non-stinging antiseptic solution (but it isn't possible to sterilize the vagina itself). A speculum is then inserted into the vagina to hold the walls apart so that the cervix (the entrance to the womb) can be seen. The cervix is steadied using a forceps-type instrument called a tenaculum. None of this will hurt, although the tenaculum may pinch momentarily. The anaesthetic is then injected into the cervix, which causes only slight pain before the area goes numb. A cannula (a slim plastic tube) is inserted through the cervix into the womb. The cannula is attached to a suction pump and the pregnancy, together with the womb lining, is simply sucked out. This procedure doesn't usually cause much discomfort, although some women experience cramping feelings in the abdomen.

When the procedure can be carried out this early, it is also known as menstrual extraction. However, the majority of terminations by vacuum suction are carried out between 7 and 12 weeks.

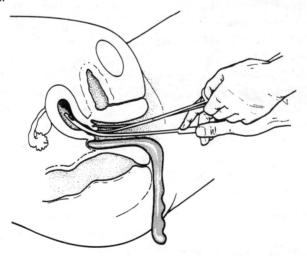

Early termination by vacuum suction: the pregnancy is removed via a slim cannula (tube). The new abortion pill – RU 486 – could be used instead. Later termination requires a wider cannula.

What happens if a termination is carried out between the 7th and 12th week of pregnancy?

The cervix needs to be dilated (widened) because larger instruments are used. A pessary containing the hormone prostaglandin may be inserted into the vagina two hours before the operation. This hormone exists naturally in the body, and one of its functions is to soften the cervix at the start of normal labour, which enables it to dilate. The pessary therefore makes the cervix easier to dilate prior to a termination.

The whole procedure can be carried out under local anaesthetic, although a general is more often used. After the anaesthetic has been given, metal or plastic rods (dilators) of increasing size are inserted into the cervix in the same way as for a D & C (dilation and curettage)*. If you are conscious, you may have cramping sensations, but dilation takes only a few minutes. The womb is then emptied using a wider cannula − the size depends on the stage of pregnancy − which is attached to a suction pump. Sometimes the womb is then gently scraped using a curette (a spoon-shaped metal instrument), alternatively any remaining tissue can be removed with small forceps.

The womb will contract back to its pre-pregnant size as the pregnancy is removed, and this can also cause cramping. You will be given synthetic oxytocin via a drip (a needle inserted in your hand or arm) or by injection to stimulate contractions and reduce bleeding. This hormone also occurs naturally in the body, causing contractions in labour.

Will I feel awful afterwards?

No. A termination by suction curettage may however leave you feeling a bit shaken physically and emotionally. You will need to spend several hours resting before leaving the hospital or clinic, especially if you've had a general anaesthetic − you may feel drowsy and sick as a result. If you're not staying overnight, you need to recover from this before going home. If possible, have someone with you who can give emotional support before and after the termination, and who can take you home.

You may continue to have cramping for a few hours after the operation and may need painkillers, but discomfort should not persist; you will have no difficulty walking. If you live alone, however, someone should be with you for at least the first night afterwards.

Will I bleed?

Yes, but you shouldn't bleed heavily. You will be wearing a sanitary towel or pad following the procedure. If you usually use tampons, make sure you have a supply of towels with you, and at home; tampons increase the risk of infection immediately after a termination and should not be used. You will be checked for bleeding before you go home, and your blood-pressure and temperature will also be taken. There may be heavier bleeding, sometimes with clots, on the third or fourth day after the operation. This is nothing to worry about, provided it doesn't persist. Bleeding to any extent should cease in about ten days, although it may continue slightly for a while longer, especially if a coil (intrauterine contraceptive device/IUCD) has been inserted at the time of termination (see page 129).

How are later terminations performed?

Dilation and Evacuation (D & E)

D & E may be carried out from 12 to about 16 weeks, i.e. in the second trimester. This is a more skilled procedure: the cervix needs dilating further, the pregnancy is larger and the womb softer. Products of conception are removed by forceps and vacuum suction under general anaesthetic. An ultrasound scan* may be needed first to confirm the size of the fetus.

Prostaglandin Induction

This is the method more often used for terminations carried out after 12 to 14 weeks. As already mentioned, the hormone prostaglandin occurs naturally in the body; it softens the cervix and stimulates contractions in labour. For termination it may be given as a vaginal pessary; more than one may be needed, given at intervals over about 24 hours. Or it can be introduced into the womb as a fluid via a tube inserted into the cervix, but this method is used less often now because more effective pessaries are available.

Alternatively, prostaglandin can be injected into the amniotic sac which surrounds the fetus. For this, the abdomen is first cleaned with antiseptic and a small area anaesthetized with a local injection. A long fine needle is then inserted through the abdomen into the womb, and may be guided by ultrasound* (you will feel pressure as the needle goes in, but no pain); the prostaglandin is then injected into the amniotic sac and the needle withdrawn.

You must be prepared for some feelings of nausea and to have diarrhoea after being give prostaglandin. Severe nausea can be relieved by taking anti-nausea drugs, or they may be given by injection.

What will I experience next?

Contractions will usually start within a few hours; these may be further stimulated by an injection of oxytocin. Painkillers will be given, either by injection or possibly via an epidural* (a spinal injection), which numbs you from the waist down. You will in effect go through a 'mini-labour'. As in normal labour, the amniotic sac will burst, releasing a gush of clear or pinkish fluid through the vagina, and contractions will continue for some hours until the pregnancy is expelled. The fetus is unlikely to be alive and independent existence would not be possible anyway. Sometimes the placenta* (afterbirth) does not come away completely, and will need removing by curette under general anaesthetic straight after the termination. Oxytocin is also given after a late termination to help the womb contract.

You have to be conscious throughout a prostaglandin termination because the procedure is too lengthy for a general anaesthetic to be safely used; it may take from 12 to 24 hours. This method is therefore more traumatic than earlier procedures. Counselling and emotional support before and after can be quite vital.

Are there any other late methods?

Hysterotomy

This procedure is used only very rarely. The fetus is removed via an incision in the abdomen, like a mini-Caesarean*. This is major surgery and is carried out only in unusual circumstances.

Why are late terminations carried out?

They are most often carried out when an amniocentesis* test has shown fetal abnormalities, such as Down's syndrome (mongolism) or the presence of genetic (hereditary) disorders. This test can be performed only after 14 weeks of pregnancy. However, a newer test called chorion villus sampling (CVS)* is sometimes an alternative and can be performed in the first trimester of pregnancy.

How long will I be in hospital after a late termination?

You will be in hospital for 24 to 48 hours after a D & E or prostaglandin abortion, so that you can be checked and monitored for any complications.

Are complications likely?

The risks are minimal when an abortion is carried out in a reputable clinic or hospital. The later the termination, however, the more likely problems are, some of which may occur a few days after the woman has left hospital.

INJURY
Injury rarely happens, but should it occur, the most likely damage is perforation of the womb by an instrument or tearing of

the cervix during dilation. Both types of damage are likely to need surgical repair at the time of termination. In the longer term, damage to the cervix may weaken it and cause a late miscarriage* in the next pregnancy. This can be corrected by placing a stitch around the cervix to support it.

INFECTION

Infection can still enter the womb, even though every care has been taken, because the vagina is not a sterile environment. Signs of this are a high temperature, severe cramping or abdominal pain, and a foul-smelling discharge, which may occur after the woman has returned home. If you have any such signs, report them to your doctor or hospital right away; infection is very serious and could affect your future fertility. It can be treated effectively with antibiotics.

PERSISTENT HEAVY BLEEDING

Haemorrhaging must also be reported to your doctor or hospital. Occasionally, tissue is left behind in the womb following a termination, causing heavy bleeding, sometimes with clots and cramps, as the womb tries to expel it. Drugs can help stimulate contractions, but if they don't work, 'retained tissue' – as it is called – can lead to infection. It will need to be removed by repeating vacuum suction or by D & C*.

It must be stressed that such problems are not the norm, and you shouldn't worry about them before a termination.

What advice can you give me on recovery?

Some women recover very quickly, particularly after an early termination, as already described. But whether you have had an early or late termination, you do need to rest for at least two days at home.

Following a late termination your stomach may feel heavy and you will bleed lightly for two to three weeks, although it may not be constant, and some women hardly bleed at all. Use sanitary towels, not tampons, until bleeding ceases. It is safe to take a shower or bath following a termination.

You may also have mild cramps for several days after a late termination. Avoid doing anything strenuous, such as heavy lifting (see page 111) for about a week, as this can make bleeding and cramps worse. As just mentioned, you must report any heavy bleeding, severe cramps or an offensive discharge to your doctor or hospital. Breast soreness, and other signs of pregnancy, may last for a week; if they go on for longer they need reporting, too.

You may feel fatigued and depressed. This can be due to altered hormonal levels, particularly following a late abortion; these will adjust in a few weeks, but there may also be psychological reasons which you might want to talk to someone about.

I would like to talk through my feelings about my termination. Where can I get help?

As with pre-abortion counselling, your doctor, family planning clinic or a pregnancy advisory service can help. Sympathetic post-abortion counselling can be just as necessary, even when the woman is relieved the termination is over. It's not at all unusual to have unresolved feelings of conflict and sadness afterwards. It may be particularly hard for a woman whose pregnancy was wanted but was ended due to circumstances beyond her control, such as fetal abnormality, or because her own health made it inadvisable.

Do I need to have a check-up following a termination if there are no problems?

Yes, definitely, even if all seems to be well. This will be arranged for four to six weeks after the procedure.

Questions Women Most Often Ask About Termination

Does an abortion always work?

Just occasionally with a very early termination the pregnancy may be missed because it is so small. If you continue to have

signs of pregnancy afterwards, another pregnancy test will be
done and the procedure repeated. Sometimes the tissue may be
sent for analysis to ensure it is normal and that the pregnancy is
not ectopic (a pregnancy outside the womb, usually in the
Fallopian tube). An ectopic pregnancy must always be terminated and different procedures are used – see Chapter 5, page 81.

Will having an abortion affect my sex life?

No, not after a well-conducted, legal abortion. If there are sexual problems, they will most likely have psychological and emotional causes affecting you and/or your partner. Counselling can
help and, if necessary, sex therapy.

When is it safe to have sex again after a termination?

It is best to wait until the bleeding ceases. If you have intercourse before that, your partner should use a condom to reduce
the risk of infection while the cervix is still open, and to prevent a further pregnancy.

Is it possible to become pregnant straight away?

Yes it is. You may not have a period for about four to six
weeks, but you will ovulate (produce a ripe egg) and this can
happen very soon after a termination. Lack of contraception, or
a method which fails, so often results in an unwanted pregnancy.
You must therefore discuss contraception with your doctor or
gynaecologist. Do this either at the time you have the termination or, if you can't face talking about it then, do so when you
have your check-up. Your partner must continue using condoms
until you decide on another effective method. If you are not in
a stable relationship, condoms are essential anyway. Don't have
sex again without contraception unless you want to become
pregnant.

How soon after a termination can I start using contraception?

AN INTRAUTERINE CONTRACEPTIVE DEVICE
The IUCD, also called the coil, can be inserted in your womb straight after an early termination and will be effective right away. Following a later termination, you need to wait until your first period to allow time for the womb to return to normal, otherwise the device might cause damage or be expelled.

THE PILL
The pill can be taken right away following an early or late termination, or you can start taking it on the first day of your next period. It will become effective after your first menstrual cycle.

A DIAPHRAGM OR CERVICAL CAP
A diaphragm or cervical cap needs to be fitted about a month after termination, when the cervix and vagina have returned to normal.

NATURAL FAMILY PLANNING METHODS
Natural methods cannot be used until your periods are regular, and this may take some months. Even then, they are not the most reliable form of contraception.

STERILIZATION*
Sterilization is a permanent method of contraception, and you will be unable to conceive again afterwards. Minor surgery is needed. It is inadvisable to be sterilized at the time of termination, unless you were already planning to have this done when the pregnancy intervened. It is inadvisable because having to undergo a termination is stressful and therefore not the best time to make a major decision about your fertility.

If I've had unprotected sex and could be pregnant, are there any ways of avoiding an abortion?

If you've had unprotected sex at the time of ovulation*, midway between your periods, it can be possible to prevent an unwanted pregnancy if you act quickly.

Having an IUCD contraceptive inserted within five days of intercourse will prevent a fertilized egg from implanting in the womb. Alternatively your doctor may prescribe the 'morning after' pill; it needs to be taken within 72 hours of intercourse. You in fact take two pills followed by two more 12 hours later. These are high-dosage contraceptive pills and can cause nausea, headaches and breast tenderness. They don't provide any lasting protection, unlike the IUCD, and you can become pregnant afterwards, even before your period. This is definitely emergency contraception and not for repeated use.

Can a pregnancy be ended in any other ways -- apart from the methods already described?

No. Resorting to old-fashioned, dangerous methods, such as gin, hot baths and throwing yourself downstairs could leave you injured and still pregnant. Never even consider having an illegal abortion. It would be expensive and is often agonizing and ineffective; your health and life could be at serious risk.

How safe is a legal abortion?

It is in fact safer than a full-term pregnancy and delivery. Even though the mortality rate in pregnancy and childbirth is low nowadays in developed countries, it is even lower for legal abortion, especially if carried out early.

Does having an abortion mean that I will have difficult pregnancies when I want children?

No, this is a myth.

Are new methods of termination being developed?

Yes. There is a new 'abortion pill'; it causes the body to expel the fetus in early pregnancy. Called RU 486, it is taken by mouth in tablet form, after which a single prostaglandin pessary is inserted into the vagina 48 hours later; the prostaglandin may cause nausea and diarrhoea. Shortly after insertion, the pregnancy aborts completely in 95 per cent of cases.

8

MISCARRIAGE

Minor surgical treatment can be necessary when there is a miscarriage − or spontaneous abortion, as it is know medically. This is unlike a termination of pregnancy*, even though the word 'abortion' is used by doctors to describe it. Miscarriage is the term used to describe a pregnancy that ends, or aborts, naturally before the 24th week. It can be a distressing experience, but knowing what to do if it happens, and understanding the treatments, can help a woman cope.

Can you explain why a pregnancy may miscarry?

The main reason for miscarriages in early pregnancy (during the first three months, or trimester) is that the fetus is not developing normally and so the body rejects it. This is not unusual, and is nothing to be alarmed about in itself; most women who miscarry find that the next pregnancy results in the birth of a normal, healthy baby.

Later miscarriages are less common. They may happen for the same reason, but more often there are other causes. The womb may be malformed or distorted by fibroids*; the cervix (the entrance to the womb) may be 'incompetent' − not strong enough to hold the pregnancy inside until full term. Such problems may be treatable, so that future pregnancies don't miscarry.

If the mother suffers from certain serious illnesses during pregnancy, the fetus may die and be expelled, but not all serious illnesses in pregnancy will cause this to happen.

How would I know if I was going to miscarry?

You may be unaware of it very early in pregnancy when there is little fetal tissue; you would have what appears to be a late period, or the miscarriage might simply occur as a blood clot. Spotting in early pregnancy may be signs of a threatened miscarriage, but this is quite common and the pregnancy often continues normally. Heavier bleeding and crampy period-like pain can also be signs of an ectopic pregnancy* (a pregnancy outside the womb, usually in the Fallopian tube); this is another reason for seeking early medical advice.

Later on, in the second trimester of pregnancy, heavy bleeding and/or severe cramping, like labour pains, mean that a miscarriage is imminent. A serious sign is if the amniotic sac, in which the fetus 'floats', bursts, releasing a gush of fluid.

If an incompetent cervix gives way rapidly, the pregnancy may be released from the womb with little discomfort: the woman just has a 'dropping' sensation as it comes away.

What should I do if I start a miscarriage?

Get medical help or go to a hospital as fast as possible; call an ambulance if necessary. Have your partner or a friend with you until your doctor or the ambulance arrives. Try to collect all the miscarriage in a clean jar; this can be distressing, but it may show whether the miscarriage was complete: the fetus, amniotic sac and placenta* (afterbirth) should all be expelled. Tests may shed light on the reason for the miscarriage.

What treatment will I receive after a miscarriage?

Most early miscarriages are complete and no medical treatment necessary. You will be given an injection of a drug which helps your womb contract. Bleeding will continue for a few days, like a period, but will gradually cease. Use sanitary towels or pads, not tampons, to reduce the risks of infection.

If bleeding and cramps continue, particularly after a late miscarriage, this will be because some tissue remains in the womb.

This is called an 'incomplete abortion'. An ERPC (evacuation of retained products of conception) is carried out; this is a simple surgical procedure, like a D&C, which gently cleans the womb.

Sometimes, however, if the fetus has died, it is not expelled (a 'missed abortion'). The signs of pregnancy cease, and a pregnancy test will become negative, but periods do not return. An ultrasound scan* will confirm this diagnosis. A missed abortion is not harmful to the woman, but treatment is needed. The pregnancy will be removed by D & C* or, if it is a late abortion, it will be necessary to induce labour by using the hormone prostaglandin, as described on page 123. Going through labour to deliver a dead fetus can be deeply upsetting, and the support of someone close to you can help you through the experience.

How long does it take to recover from a miscarriage?

Physical recovery after an early miscarriage is swift. You need to rest at home for a few days, but should be fully recovered within about a week, and sometimes sooner. After a later miscarriage light bleeding may continue for longer and your stomach may feel heavy.

Avoid doing anything which could strain your abdomen for the first week (i.e. no heavy lifting, no driving). If you lost a lot of blood during the miscarriage, you will feel tired and full recovery may take two to three weeks. A blood transfusion* will be given if necessary, or iron and vitamin tablets prescribed to counteract anaemia. But psychological recovery can be just as important, if not more so, when a wanted pregnancy has ended.

The loss of our much-wanted baby has left us feeling terrible. How can we cope?

Miscarriage of a wanted pregnancy can cause intense disappointment, grief and a sense of failure in one or both partners. You may still feel pregnant, especially after a late miscarriage, and this can last a few weeks until your hormone levels adjust.

These feelings can make the miscarriage more difficult to accept, and the hormonal changes in themselves cause depression. Tell your doctor or hospital; s/he or they can put you in touch with a counsellor or support group. Counselling, and talking things through with other people who have experienced this loss, can be very helpful in enabling you and your partner to come to terms with what has happened. It can also encourage you to try for a pregnancy again.

How soon is it safe to try for another baby following a miscarriage?

You should wait until the bleeding stops before having sex again, but don't try for a pregnancy until you have had two periods.

What are my chances of having a successful pregnancy after a miscarriage?

As said at the start of the chapter, they are very good. The majority of women – about 80 per cent – have a successful pregnancy when they next try.

Questions Women Most Often Ask About Miscarriage

Are there any treatments which can prevent a miscarriage?

If you have slight bleeding and cramps early in pregnancy you may be advised to rest in bed, although it's not proven that this helps. When bleeding continues, or is heavy, at any stage in pregnancy, a pelvic examination* can be done to find out if the womb is the right size for the stage of pregnancy. An ultrasound scan* may also be carried out to check if the pregnancy is normal and the fetus alive. There are no specific treatments which can prevent a miscarriage, except when the cervix shows signs of opening (incompetence).

How is an incompetent cervix treated?

By putting a stitch in it to hold it closed, rather like a purse-string. This is called a Shirodkar suture, after the doctor who devised it, and the procedure is known as cervical cerclage. It is done in hospital under general anaesthetic and requires a 48-hour stay. A woman who has miscarried because of an incompetent cervix should have this stitch inserted at the 14th week of future pregnancies. It isn't infallible, but it does often work. The stitch is removed at 38 weeks, after which labour can be induced, or may occur naturally.

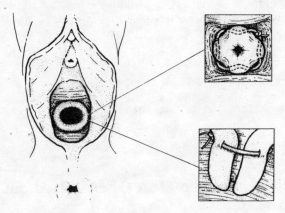

When the cervix (the entrance to the womb) is not strong enough to retain a pregnancy, this 'purse-string' stitch (a Shirodkar suture) can be inserted to hold it closed.

What other ways are there of dealing with problems leading to a miscarriage?

When a miscarriage has occurred for other reasons, tests can find the cause and future miscarriages may be preventable. For instance, a type of X-ray* called a hysterosalpingogram* can show if the womb is normal. Surgery can sometimes resolve problems caused by malformation of the womb or by fibroids*. Tests can be done for hormonal problems or genetic (hereditary) disorders which can cause miscarriage. Hormone treatment may be possible, and if there are genetic disorders the couple may be helped by genetic counselling.

Is there anything a woman can do herself to guard against having a miscarriage?

Miscarriages generally occur for reasons beyond the woman's control. However, too much alcohol (more than two small drinks a day) may increase the risk; a woman who has already miscarried may therefore be advised not to drink during pregnancy. There is also evidence that smoking increases the risk of miscarriage and fetal abnormalities because it affects the baby's growth. Smoking is a danger to health in so many ways that giving it up for good is the only sensible answer.

Could a woman or her partner unknowingly do something which causes her to miscarry?

Following a miscarriage, a couple can get the distressing idea that it had something to do with their own behaviour and must therefore be their fault, but this is almost always untrue. It's very difficult to dislodge a healthy pregnancy accidentally. Women, and their partners, often worry that having sex during pregnancy will start a miscarriage. Similarly, women also worry about taking exercise. Neither are harmful to the pregnancy, and you can continue with them for as long as you wish.

9

STERILIZATION

Sterilization ends a woman's ability to conceive. It is intended to be a permanent method of contraception, after which you will no longer be able to have children. Although skilled surgery is involved, the procedures which can be used are minor and recovery swift. The male version – called a vasectomy – is much simpler and even quicker. In this chapter we describe the operations, to give you a clear idea of what exactly this major step involves.

While this is a book primarily for women, the need for sterilization is often a partnership concern. Emotional and practical aspects which it could be helpful for you to discuss together and with your doctor are included. Whether it is you or your partner who is considering being sterilized, you must be certain the right decision is made. This will enable you to feel positive about any surgery you decide to have.

How does sterilization prevent pregnancy?

In women, the purpose of sterilization is to prevent the man's sperm and the woman's egg from meeting so that fertilization, and a pregnancy, cannot take place. In men, a vasectomy prevents the sperm from being carried in the semen, so that when a man ejaculates there are no sperm in his semen and, again, fertilization cannot happen.

What is the first step in performing a sterilization?

Starting with female sterilization, there are several methods of carrying this out. All of them stop the passage of ripe eggs down the Fallopian tubes, where fertilization takes place, before a pregnancy is started in the womb. Sterilization involves techniques which tie, sever, constrict or crush the Fallopian tubes. These are almost always carried out under general anaesthetic in hospital.

Before the surgeon can perform a sterilization, the tubes need to be brought into view. The most usual way of doing this is via a laparoscope*. The abdomen is first inflated with harmless gas to make the procedure possible. The laparoscope (a viewing instrument) is inserted via a very small incision just below the navel, and the surgical instruments used in sterilization are inserted through another very small incision near the pubic hairline (see the illustration on page 16).

Could you describe how a female sterilization is carried out using a laparoscope?

When the surgeon has the tubes in view, a sterilization can be performed as follows.

- Constriction rings made of silastic (stretchable plastic) can simply be placed over a loop made in each tube, constricting it at the base; or
- Clips made of metal or plastic can be applied to each tube in one or two places, crushing it flat so it is blocked.

Rings or clips are left permanently in place on the tubes. The method which is used depends on the surgeon's technique and experience.

How long do these procedures take?

They both take only about 15 to 20 minutes to perform. However, as a sterilization by laparoscopy is most often done under general anaesthetic, it may involve an overnight stay in hospital. But if it can be carried out early in the morning, it may be possible to do it on a day-patient basis, and you can go home in the evening. Chapter 2 on Preparing for Surgery advises on what you need to do before having a procedure under general anaesthetic.

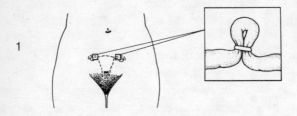

Constriction rings (1) or clips (2) are placed on the Fallopian tubes to prevent sperm and egg meeting for fertilization. Only two tiny scars are left on the abdomen following this procedure.

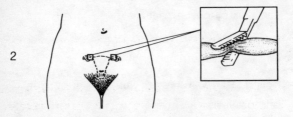

Will I feel awful afterwards?

You won't feel all that bright straight after the operation. You'll have the usual feelings following any procedure carried out by laparoscopy*. Sterilization will leave your abdomen feeling bruised: some women describe it as feeling like they've been dealt 'a kick in the stomach'. Sometimes painkillers are injected directly into the tubes during surgery to prevent this discomfort, otherwise they will be given afterwards. Arrange for someone to take you home, and allow yourself a few days to recover.

Are all female sterilizations done by laparoscopy?

About 90 per cent of all female sterilizations are now done by laparoscopy. It may not be possible if the woman is very overweight or has adhesions (scar tissue) from previous abdominal surgery. In these cases a procedure called a mini-laparotomy would more likely be used. This is an incision of about 5 cm (2 in), or less, which is made just above the pubic hairline. A tubal ligation can then be performed.

This involves lifting a loop of each tube in turn, tying it at the base with a soluble stitch, and then cutting off the top of the loop, which removes about 3 cm (1½ in) of each tube. The cut ends heal over and drift apart. Alternatively, rings or clips may be placed on the tubes, as during a sterilization by laparoscopy.

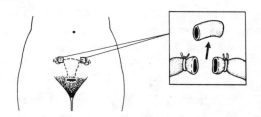

Tubal ligation involves tying and removing a section of each Fallopian tube via a small incision in the lower abdomen.

If a sterilization is carried out following childbirth, a mini-laparotomy incision is made just below the navel, because at this time the womb and tubes are elevated in the abdomen. But immediately after childbirth is generally not the best time to be sterilized (more on this later).

How would I feel after a mini-laparotomy, and how long does recovery take?

This is a more extensive procedure than a sterilization by laparoscopy. The abdominal soreness could be described as more like two kicks in the stomach, except that you will be given painkillers, so won't have to suffer.

You'll be in hospital for about three days and may need a drip (a needle inserted in a vein in your hand or arm through which fluid lost during surgery is replaced). You may also need a catheter (a tube in your urethra to help you urinate), but this is by no means always the case.

If the stitches in your abdomen are non-soluble, they will be removed after about five days – this can be done either on a return visit to the hospital or by your own doctor. Rest for about a week and avoid heavy lifting (see pages 111–12) for two to three weeks.

Are there any other ways of performing a sterilization?

There is a procedure which is carried out through an incision in the top of the vagina, called a colpotomy. The tubes are pulled to the incision and then either tied and severed or have clips/rings applied, as already described. This method is very uncommon now because the risks of infection afterwards are greater, since the vagina is not a sterile environment.

Another sterilization technique, which is also uncommon now, uses diathermy (electrical heat) to burn through and seal the tubes. With this method there is the danger that the heat generated will damage other internal organs.

Methods using a hysteroscope* (an instrument for viewing inside the womb) are in an experimental stage at the time of writing. These involve ways of blocking the tubes from inside the womb, but so far have not proved very successful.

Can a sterilization be carried out during another operation?

If the abdomen is being opened for a more extensive operation, such as a Caesarean birth* (the baby is delivered via an abdominal incision), sterilization can be carried out at the same time. This is often advised after a third Caesarean delivery, because each successive Caesarean is liable to increase slightly the risk of complications.

Of course, if a hysterectomy* (removal of the womb) is necessary to treat a disorder, this would result in sterility. And if the tubes and ovaries are removed, either during a hysterectomy or separately, this will also end fertility. But such major surgery would not be carried out only as a sterilization procedure these days.

Is female sterilization immediately effective?

Yes. You will not be able to conceive after the operation. It is safe to have sexual intercourse as soon as you feel able.

What happens in a male sterilization?

A vasectomy also involves severing two tubes. These tubes are called the vas deferens. They carry sperm from the testes to the base of the penis where the sperm joins the semen before ejaculation. The operation is much simpler and quicker than a female sterilization because the male scrotum (which contains the tubes and the testes) is outside the body, unlike the woman's Fallopian tubes. A vasectomy is done under local anaesthetic at a family planning clinic or hospital out-patient department.

The operation takes less than half an hour. A tiny incision is made on one side of the scrotum and the vas deferens is pulled through it in a loop. Usually, a section of the loop is cut out and the ends sealed with soluble stitches; the ends may be bent back on themselves and tied again. Diathermy (heat) may be used to seal the ends rather than stitches. The severed ends are then pushed back into the scrotum and the incision stitched together with soluble stitches. The same procedure is repeated on the other side of the scrotum.

There will be some bruising and soreness afterwards, and the man should not attempt to drive himself home; he will need someone else to do this. He should take it easy for a day or two and wear tight underpants or an athletic support for the next two weeks. Complications are unusual, but if there is any inflammation or discharge from the incision, this needs to be reported to the doctor. Both can be treated with antibiotics.

Is a vasectomy immediately effective, like a female sterilization?

No. Sperm will continue to be present in the semen for a time. Contraception will still be needed until two consecutive samples of semen tested contain no sperm. This is usually the case after about 30 ejaculations, and semen samples will be needed for testing then. Semen production, and sexual performance, are unaffected by the operation. Intercourse, with contraception, can be resumed soon after the operation, usually in about a week. Of course, the more often ejaculation takes place, the sooner the operation will be effective.

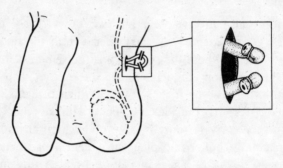

In a vasectomy, the vas deferens (sperm-carrying tubes) are pulled through tiny incisions each side of the scrotum. These tubes are then tied and severed.

Where do the sperm go after a vasectomy?

They are still produced in the testes but, as they are no longer carried in the semen, the body reabsorbs them with no ill-effects.

What advice can you give on which partner should be sterilized?

As said at the start of the chapter, whether it is you or your partner who is considering being sterilized, you must be certain you make the right decision. Sterilization is a method of last resort, and the decision to be sterilized should never be rushed or made under stress.

The first thing to do is to see your doctor or visit your family planning clinic. Although a partner's consent to the operation is not officially required, it is best if you are counselled together. It will be most helpful if you and your partner can discuss the matter with a doctor who is experienced in family planning.

Even though a vasectomy is the simpler operation, more female sterilizations are carried out because it is the woman who bears the children and most often takes responsibility for contraception. Men are inclined to worry about the effects a vasectomy will have on their masculinity and virility, although such fears are in fact groundless. Reassurance from other men who have had vasectomies can help to remove these fears.

As for a woman, a man should only consider being sterilized if he is certain he will never want any more children under any circumstances. But this can be a very complex matter. Some people value their fertility as part of their self-image and could feel they have 'lost' an important part of themselves after a sterilization, even though they have no wish to reproduce. Neither of you should have a sterilization simply to please the other partner – you must be sure it will also be right for you personally.

If I want to be sterilized, what other emotional and practical aspects would it be helpful for me to consider and discuss?

Your doctor or family planning clinic can refer you to a gynaecologist for a female sterilization. S/he will need to be sure that your reasons for wanting a sterilization fully justify the operation, and that you are psychologically ready for it. If you have a partner, as is likely in this situation, it is certainly a good idea for him to visit them with you, as already mentioned.

Some of the following emotional and practical aspects may be relevant to your life, and some could also apply to a partner who is considering sterilization.

- You have completed your family and other methods of contraception you have tried are unreliable or unacceptable (for example, perhaps you have come off the pill and are finding it difficult to use another method).

  If you and your children are still young, you must consider the possibility that you might lose a child and perhaps want another. This is also a reason why female sterilization immediately after childbirth is not a good idea.

  Should your relationship with your partner end through separation or death, might you want a child with another partner?

Maybe you have had an unwanted pregnancy, and perhaps a termination* (an abortion). The decision to have a
termination is often traumatic in itself, and it may be
inadvisable to consider ending your fertility at the same
time as having a termination.

However, if you are in a stable relationship and have a
family who are growing up, sterilization may be the best
answer. But where one partner is much younger than the
other, the older partner may be advised to have the operation.

- Health reasons.

If, for instance, a genetic (hereditary) disorder affects
one or both partners and could be passed to children,
sterilization can be a very sensible option. But if, deep
down, there is still the desire to have a child, sterilization
may not be right for you or your partner. Have you had
genetic counselling? Your doctor or family planning clinic
can put you in touch with a counsellor.

Similarly, if you have a health problem which could be
made worse by childbearing, sterilization may be the
answer. In certain cases, however, it may still be possible
to have a child if the pregnancy is carefully managed.

Also, medical progress may change such situations and
you may want to consider this possibility in relation to
your own wishes.

- Economic reasons.

You need to ask yourself if you might want to change
your mind if your life were different. Things may get better. How would you feel then?

- You are sure you never want children.

Increasingly, requests which are made for this reason
are given a sympathetic hearing and discussed in terms of
what would suit you as a person.

- You hope it will improve a difficult relationship.

Sterilization alone cannot improve a relationship which
is in difficulty sexually or emotionally. Your doctor or
family planning clinic can again help by putting you in
touch with a relationship counsellor.

- There is one further aspect which is seldom mentioned in books, but which can have a profound influence in the long term: some people come from a religious background where sterilization, like abortion, is condemned. If this is the case with you or your partner, you may need to come to terms with it before having a sterilization.

These considerations are not meant to give the impression that sterilization should be an obstacle course, but it is wise to think and talk through every aspect of your situation. If you have any doubts, it is certainly worth persevering with other methods of contraception, and seeking help and advice on these from your doctor or family planning clinic; see also the References and Further Reading section of this book.

Might I be refused a sterilization?

If it was thought not to be in your best interests you would be advised against it. The most common reason for this advice is probably on the grounds of 'being too young'. However, a doctor may see 'obstetric' age (i.e. how many children a woman has already) as being more important than her actual age. For instance, a woman of 23 who has already had three children might in fact be seen as a better candidate for sterilization than a woman of 33 who has not yet had any. Whatever the reason given for this advice, you would still have the right to go to a different doctor or ask to be referred to another gynaecologist, if you disagreed with it.

Questions Women Most Often Ask About Sterilization

Can a sterilization be reversed?

No one should ever be sterilized with this in mind. Skilled microsurgical techniques can often restore the Fallopian tubes, but it requires a full operation through the abdomen, is difficult to perform and carries no guarantee of success. It is least difficult to carry out if clips were used, but as already stated, reversal is a more extensive procedure than the original sterilization. Afterwards the chances of pregnancy may be no greater than 50 per cent, and the risk of an ectopic pregnancy* (the fertilized egg lodging in the tube, preventing the pregnancy from continuing) is increased.

A vasectomy can sometimes be reversed by rejoining the vas deferens. Again, this is a more extensive operation, but it is simpler than a female sterilization reversal. The chances of parenthood are also reduced afterwards.

The vast majority of requests for sterilization reversals come from people who have formed new partnerships and were sterilized during a previous relationship. This is why it is very important to consider this possibility before being sterilized.

If a sterilization cannot be reversed, are there any ways round the problem?

It may be possible for a woman to have in vitro fertilization (IVF)*. For this procedure ripe eggs are removed directly from her ovaries, fertilized outside her body by mixing them with her partner's sperm, and then placed in her womb. This bypasses the tubes. The success rate of this technique is still low, and it is not widely available. Before a vasectomy, a man could have some of his sperm frozen and kept in a sperm bank for possible future use in artificial insemination*.

Does sterilization often fail?

No. In women the overall failure rate is about 1 in 500; in women over 40 it will be less than this. In men it is only about 1 in 1,000. Every care will be taken to ensure that no pregnancy already exists at the time of sterilization. If there is any doubt, a pregnancy test will be carried out. It is likely anyway that a D & C (dilation and curettage)*, which removes the womb lining, will be done as a general health check during a female sterilization. This will prevent any pregnancy. A sterilization is most likely to fail if carried out immediately after childbirth, which is another reason against doing it at this time.

Why does sterilization fail?

It may fail because rings or clips occasionally come adrift and
the crushed tubes regenerate; the natural movement of organs in
the pelvis may be responsible for this. Sometimes even severed
Fallopian tubes simply rejoin spontaneously. Similarly, in men
the vas deferens may occasionally rejoin of their own accord. In
women, the increased blood flow to the pelvic organs during
pregnancy may be a reason why sterilization is more likely to
fail when carried out after childbirth: the tubes have a greater
ability to regenerate then.

If my sterilization failed, would I have any legal redress?

Before the operation, you would be asked to sign a consent
form which should say that it cannot be guaranteed 100 per
cent successful; this is so even when it is carried out correctly.
You would therefore need to prove that the operation had been
carried out negligently.

Is there a foolproof method of sterilization?

For women, the more extensive the procedure, the less likely it is
to fail. Removing the tubes altogether (bilateral salpingectomy) is
more certain to be successful than clipping or tying them. This
may be carried out after a woman has had several Caesarean
deliveries, or as a re-sterilization if another method has failed. In
men, the only foolproof method would be castration (removal of
both testes), and no one would seriously recommend that!

Would I continue to have periods after sterilization?

Yes. Your ovaries would continue to produce ripe eggs and you
would still have a menstrual cycle. Some women find that their
periods become heavier after sterilization. This has not been definitely linked to the operation. It may occur because the woman
has come off the pill; periods are lighter on the pill. As women
grow older, periods can become heavier anyway.

What happens to the eggs produced by the ovaries? Where do they go when they can no longer pass down the tubes?

They are reabsorbed by the body with no ill-effects, just as a man's sperm is after a vasectomy. There's no need to worry about an 'egg mountain'!

Are there any long-term problems after sterilization?

No. Any problems, such as infection, are likely to arise soon after surgery, and can be treated.

What effects will sterilization have on my sex life?

It won't have any adverse effects. You will be free from worry about contraception and an unwanted pregnancy. A sterilization which is the result of a well-considered decision can make a good sexual relationship even better.

10

POLYPS

It's simple to remove polyps from inside the womb or from the cervical canal (the entrance to the womb). A polyp is a lump attached to a stalk which either grows from the membrane that lines the womb or from the cervix. Polyps can grow singly or in groups, and vary in size from very small to the size of a grape or even larger sometimes. Although they are almost always benign, and not serious in themselves, they can cause symptoms which need investigating by minor surgery.

How can I tell if I have polyps in my womb?

You can't always tell. Small polyps in the womb may cause no problems and so don't need treatment, but larger ones, or groups, can produce symptoms. If you have heavy, irregular periods, or any bleeding between periods, or if you have a vaginal discharge, particularly if it is blood-stained, you must see your doctor. These symptoms can be due to polyps, but may have other causes which also need investigating (see Chapter 1 on Diagnosing Women's Problems).

I've noticed that I bleed during and after intercourse, and am worried about this. Could it be due to polyps?

Yes, it could. Polyps which protrude from the cervix can be damaged by thrusting during intercourse, causing them to bleed. If bleeding is due to polyps, it's easy for your doctor to diagnose them by doing a routine pelvic examination*: they are red-tipped and can be seen easily. But again, you must report any bleeding during and/or after sex to your doctor promptly, because it is important to find out whether or not polyps are the cause.

What will be done about my symptoms, and can I be sure that all polyps will be removed?

If your symptoms could be due to polyps in the womb, they will be investigated by D & C (dilation and curettage)*, possibly coupled with hysteroscopy*. A hysteroscope is a small telescope with a light at one end, which allows the surgeon to look inside the womb before and after D & C. This simple surgical procedure is done under general anaesthetic and requires at the most an overnight stay in hospital. Many women go home the same day.

The polyp(s) and samples of the womb lining are removed for examination, so the procedure is both an investigation and a treatment. There may be mild cramping pains and some bleeding for a day or two afterwards. Sanitary towels need to be worn rather than tampons, because tampons increase the risk of infection.

Polyps which protrude from the cervix can sometimes be removed in the out-patient clinic. This is done by twisting them off using forceps, which is virtually painless and doesn't require an anaesthetic. But if they are large or numerous, removal may need to be done in hospital under general anaesthetic.

Questions Women Most Often Ask About Polyps

Why have I got polyps?

The reason isn't known, but they are quite common and can occur at any age, although they are less common after the menopause. They are not something which affect women only: sometimes they grow in the nose, throat and bowel of men and women alike. But in women they may occasionally be a sign of fibroids when they are present in the womb, in which case there is likely to be heavy and/or irregular bleeding. Fibroids are also benign growths, but – unlike polyps – they develop in the muscular wall of the womb (see Chapter 11 for further information).

I've had some polyps removed. Will they regrow?

It is possible, but if they did recur, they would be new polyps rather than old ones which have regrown. People who have had polyps seem to have a tendency to get them again, but if this happens, they are always easy to treat if necessary.

Do polyps make it difficult to become pregnant?

Almost certainly not, unless they are of the fibroid variety, i.e. growing out from the muscular wall of the womb. These types of polyps often grow larger than simple polyps, and so occupy more space within the womb. Cervical polyps would be most unlikely to affect conception or the subsequent pregnancy.

I've heard that polyps can be cancerous. Is this true?

It is extremely rare for polyps in the womb or on the cervix to become malignant, but it is always advisable to have them removed if they are causing any of the problems we have described.

11

FIBROIDS

It isn't really known why some women develop these benign tumours of the womb, but about a quarter of all women have fibroids by the time they are in their 40s. Often no treatment is required, although surgery to remove them is sometimes necessary. The type of operation can depend on the woman's particular needs, so if you have fibroids, your doctor should discuss these with you. Here we explain the options and how surgery can relieve symptoms or restore fertility.

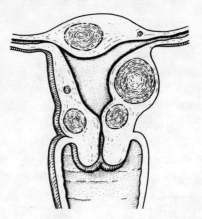

Large fibroids can necessitate a myomectomy — an operation which removes the fibroids only — or a hysterectomy, to remove the entire womb.

You say that fibroids are benign tumours. What does this mean, and how serious are they?

Fibroids are non-cancerous growths, which means they are not dangerous in themselves: they do not invade surrounding tissue or spread like cancer. They are made of fibrous and muscular tissue. Usually, there is more than one. They develop in the muscular wall of the womb (uterus), as illustrated, and can grow out from the wall into the cavity of the womb; they may also occur along the cervical canal, but this is rare. The size of fibroids is often compared to fruit and vegetables, because they can range from pea-sized through tomato and orange to very large: grapefruit- or melon-sized. There can be several which all vary in size, but if any grow large they can cause discomfort and other unpleasant symptoms, as described below.

How will I know if I have fibroids?

You may not know. Sometimes they are only discovered during a route gynaecological check: they may be felt during a bi-manual pelvic examination*. But if fibroids distort the inside of the womb (the cavity) they can cause heavy, irregular periods, with blood clots and cramping pains. Fibroids may increase the number of blood vessels in the wall of the womb, making bleeding heavier. There may also be bleeding between periods, although this is less common. Large fibroids can press on the bladder and bowel, resulting in the urge to urinate frequently, constipation and backache. If they put pressure on the veins from the legs, they can aggravate varicose veins. You may be able to feel a large fibroid by pressing on your abdomen, but this is not always the case. A slim woman with very large fibroids may be aware that her abdomen is more rounded than it was, but there is a lot of room in the pelvis, so they may not be obvious.

I'm having difficulty becoming pregnant. Could this be because I have fibroids which need to be removed?

It might be. If fibroids block the Fallopian tubes, you will not become pregnant because the egg cannot be fertilized (see page 47). And if the inside of the womb (the cavity) is distorted by fibroids, or the womb has become very large due to fibroids, it will not be able to support a pregnancy. But fibroids do not often cause infertility, so there may be other reasons why you are having difficulty in becoming pregnant – see Chapter 4 on Investigating and Treating Infertility.

I'm told I have some quite small fibroids which do not need treatment, but my doctor wants to check them from time to time. Does this mean I may need to have treatment, and if so, what will be done?

Treatment is unnecessary if your fibroids are small and not causing you any problems – and this is frequently the case with fibroids – but your doctor will want to check their size from time to time. If they ever do cause trouble, such as heavy periods, you will be referred to a gynaecologist. After examining you, s/he may carry out an ultrasound scan* to show the size and position of the fibroids. A blood test may also be done to find out whether heavy periods are making you anaemic (you may be feeling tired and 'low'). Heavy periods are sometimes helped by taking hormone tablets. But if this does not work, or fibroids are causing other problems, treatment will depend on your age and desire to have children.

An examination by hysteroscope* – a viewing instrument which allows a direct look inside the womb – will show whether heavy periods are being caused by small fibroids growing into the cavity (these may also affect fertility). If so, they could be removed individually by resectoscope (as illustrated), enabling you to retain your fertility. This simple procedure can be carried out under local or general anaesthetic on a day-patient basis.

If you don't wish to remain fertile, these small fibroids could be treated by full endometrial resection* or ablation*, minor procedures which remove the entire womb lining permanently, and the fibroids with it. It is the womb lining, or endometrium, which is shed as a period, so if it no longer exists, heavy periods will cease.

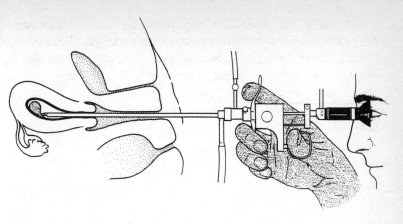

Small fibroids which grow into the cavity of the womb can be removed simply by resectoscope.

A hysterectomy* will be recommended for other types of troublesome fibroids. This removes them all with the womb. Chapter 15 on Hysterectomy gives details of this major operation and advice on recovery. But if you wish to have children, or simply want to retain your womb, perhaps to 'keep your options open', these fibroids can be removed by an operation called a myomectomy (the medical name for fibroids being myomata).

Is it true that a myomectomy is a bigger operation than a hysterectomy?

Sometimes it can be, but this depends on the size, position and number of fibroids. Each fibroid needs to be 'shelled out' individually and the womb returned to its normal shape and size. This may mean a longer operation than a hysterectomy, where the womb itself is completely removed. However, a myomectomy can be quite straightforward.

Can a myomectomy always be done?

If the womb is very much misshapen by fibroids, so that it could be extremely difficult to restore to its normal size and function, the surgeon may want to reserve the right to do a hysterectomy if necessary. Your permission for this will be asked before the operation, and the surgeon should discuss it with you. A hysterectomy is rarely needed, however.

I will be having a myomectomy. What advice can you give me on preparing for surgery and on recovery afterwards?

Preparing for a myomectomy is much the same as for any other operation carried out under general anaesthetic in hospital. Chapter 2 on Preparing for Surgery will help you. But there are some aspects of preparation which it is worth repeating here.

1. Check the dates when your periods are due, to ensure that you will not be menstruating at the time of surgery.
2. Because this is an abdominal operation, involving an incision over the womb – along the top of your pubic hair – the hair needs to be removed. This makes some women feel vulnerable because it changes their intimate appearance. But the hair does grow again quite fast, and will hide the scar, which will gradually fade anyway.
3. When you come round from the anaesthetic you may be on a drip* (given via a needle inserted into a vein in your hand or arm). This replaces fluid lost during surgery; you may need a blood transfusion* too, which is given in the same way. This is painless but not very pleasant; it is soon over, though.
4. You will feel sore – 'as if my abdomen has been bruised' is how one patient described it – or the area around the incision under the dressing may be numb. You will be wearing a sanitary towel, but it is unlikely that you will bleed heavily. A catheter (a tube) may be inserted into your urethra to help you pass urine, although this is not always necessary.
5. You can expect to be in hospital for about a week, and will be out of bed and walking around within a day or two. This is, of course, to prevent blood clots forming in your legs as a result of inactivity.
6. The stitches in the incision will be removed before you leave hospital. This won't hurt at all if done carefully.

Your womb may have been stitched with soluble catgut; as the stitches dissolve, you may feel slight tingling sensations. If surgery was carried out by laser (a powerful beam of infra-red light used for cutting), stitches in the womb are not needed.

7. You won't feel too good for about three or four weeks after the operation. You should be able to walk without feeling you 'have to be careful' within that time. But take things easy. Don't do anything strenuous or go back to work before then.

8. Your stomach muscles may have become slack after surgery, so it will help if you do some exercises to strengthen them (see page 211), but wait first for about four weeks.

9. Some women can feel very depressed after a myomectomy (or indeed any major operation) simply because it is a physical and emotional shock to the system. But with a myomectomy, your womb has been returned to normal and this in itself can be a source of relief and happiness.

Questions Women Most Often Ask About Fibroids

Is there any way I could have avoided getting fibroids?

No, there is no way of knowing whether they will develop. But they are more common in women who have had no children, or who had children later in life. You are therefore less likely to develop them if you had children while still in your teens or 20s.

They are also associated with high levels of the hormone oestrogen, which plays a vital part in the menstrual cycle. Levels of this hormone drop during and after the menopause when periods stop, and so fibroids are likely to shrink – or disappear, if they are small – at this time.

I've had a myomectomy. Will the fibroids grow again?

There is a small risk of this happening, although if you're near-ing the menopause the chances are reduced. If fibroids do recur, and cause unpleasant symptoms, a hysterectomy* (removal of the womb) is likely to be advised, rather than another myomec-tomy.

When can I have sex again after a myomectomy?

The womb needs time to heal, so you should wait for about six weeks, but lovemaking without penetration is perfectly safe, and can also be very reassuring during convalescence.

How soon can I try for a baby after having my fibroids removed?

It depends on the extent of surgery – your gynaecologist will advise you. A minimum wait of three months is likely – and sometimes six months is preferable – to ensure that your womb has healed and that you'll have a good chance of becoming pregnant.

I know I have fibroids, and I've had some bleeding between periods. Should I have a check-up, or is it safe to assume that it is due to them?

You should have a check-up. There can be other causes of bleeding between periods, and your doctor may want to ensure that your fibroids are the cause and not something else. You may need a D & C (dilation and curettage)*, which is a simple surgical procedure used to remove the womb lining for exami-nation. If the bleeding is due to polyps – see Chapter 10 – they can be removed during the D & C.

Are there any risks if I become pregnant while I have fibroids?

There are usually none if your fibroids are small. However, the blood supply to a fibroid may be affected, in which case the fibroid will degenerate. This can cause you some pain. But unless your fibroids are large or numerous, there should not be any risk to the actual pregnancy.

Will my fibroids ever become malignant?

This is extremely unlikely. Just very occasionally a large fibroid may turn into a cancerous tumour, called a sarcoma, but it would probably have caused symptoms before then and you would have had it removed.

12

OVARIAN TUMOURS

Tumours of the ovaries can be either benign or malignant (cancerous). The vast majority are benign, and can be surgically removed if necessary, but ovarian tumours are usually symptomless in their early stages, just when surgery for cancer can be most successful. This is a major reason why it is so important to have regular check-ups, particularly if you are over 40, because the chances of malignancy increase with age.

What exactly are ovarian tumours?

There are several different types of tumours. They may be cystic (fluid-filled) or solid. Whether they are benign or malignant, they very often have both liquid and solid contents, although benign tumours are most often cystic rather than solid.

The most common kind of benign tumour is called a **functional cyst**. This is because these cysts occur when the ovary producing a ripe egg during the monthly cycle fails to function properly. Why this sometimes happens is not clear, but the result is that the follicle (or small capsule) in the ovary where the egg grows fails to burst and release the ripe egg at ovulation*. Instead, the cavity, which is already filled with fluid, over-expands to form a blister-like cyst.

Functional cysts may also occur after ovulation in the yellow tissue (called the corpus luteum, or 'yellow body') which then forms from the follicle. It's possible to have more than one such cyst, and they can occur on either ovary or both.

Small functional cysts (less than 5 cm/2 in) often go away without treatment. Larger ones, and other types of tumour, don't do this, and surgery is needed to remove them.

There is a not uncommon benign condition called **polycystic ovaries**. The ovaries are slightly enlarged by multiple pea-sized cysts. This is due to a hormonal imbalance*, which can sometimes be treated successfully by drugs. If this doesn't work, however, surgery is needed.

Other types of tumour are the result of abnormal cell growth (which isn't necessarily cancerous) and, as already mentioned, will require surgical removal. These include **serous cysts**, which contain watery fluid, but – unlike functional cysts – the casing of the cyst is made up of abnormal cells. **Mucinous cysts** contain jelly-like fluid. The ovaries have the potential to create fetal tissue from which a baby develops: **dermoid cysts** contain this tissue. Blood-filled **endometriotic cysts** are also called 'chocolate cysts' because their contents resemble chocolate sauce. They occur as part of endometriosis*, the disorder where fragments of the womb lining (the endometrium) are present outside the womb, in the pelvis, where they cause painful inflammation, particularly during periods.

The causes of abnormal cell growth tumours are unknown. The majority are benign, but the serous and mucinous types are prone to malignant change.

Do cysts ever cause symptoms?

Small cysts are usually 'silent', unless they are functional cysts, which may cause irregular and often too-frequent periods. If a small cyst causes pain, it means that something has happened to it. There may be bleeding into the cyst (a haemorrhage), the cyst fluid may be leaking out into the pelvis, or the whole ovary may have twisted, cutting off its own blood supply. Medical help is then urgently needed.

With the polycystic ovary condition, women frequently have sparse periods, put on weight and may notice increased growth of body hair. They may also be having difficulty conceiving.

Some cysts, especially the mucinous type, may become large

and put pressure on the bowel or bladder, causing constipation
or frequency of urination. They may even cause a visible
swelling in the abdomen similar to pregnancy. Menstrual distur-
bance of any kind is often a late symptom.

*What about malignant tumours: are there any symptoms a woman would be
able to recognize?*

Because both benign and malignant tumours are usually 'silent'
in their early stages, a woman has no way of knowing whether
she has a malignant ovarian tumour. By the time she has symptoms, cancer may be advanced. Even then, symptoms are vague.
There may be abdominal discomfort, wind, stomach upsets,
nausea and abdominal swelling due to fluid produced by the
cancerous ovary (no one knows why this happens).
Unfortunately, women sometimes only discover that they have
ovarian cancer when they see their doctor because they want to
lose weight: their clothes are becoming too tight. In fact, they
are not getting fatter; it's simply the result of the fluid build-up.
Abnormal vaginal bleeding (i.e. any bleeding which is out of
the ordinary) may sometimes occur as a symptom. But there is
absolutely no need for things to get this serious if a woman has
regular check-ups.

How does the doctor diagnose ovarian tumours?

Most are found during a routine bi-manual pelvic examination*.
In their normal state the ovaries are about the size of walnuts. A
tumour can be felt as a swelling of the ovary.

What would be done if an enlarged ovary were found?

This would depend on your age. A woman under 40 who
appeared to have a small cyst (or cysts) would probably have a
further check-up four to eight weeks later, after one or two of
her monthly cycles, to see if it has disappeared spontaneously,
as would very likely happen. If it were still there then, further
investigation would be needed.

Malignant tumours are rare in younger women, but in a woman over 40 any ovarian enlargement needs prompt investigation because, as said at the start of this chapter, the chances of malignancy increase with age.

How are these investigation carried out?

An ultrasound scan* will show the size and position of the cyst(s). It will also reveal to what extent the contents are fluid or solid. A dermoid cyst may show up on an X-ray*. Usually, however, diagnostic surgery is needed to decide on any treatment needed. This can be done by laparoscopy* – a minor surgical procedure carried out under general anaesthetic in hospital, which requires at most an overnight stay. Laparoscopy allows the ovaries to be viewed directly. Tissue samples can be removed and analysed straight away to find out whether they are benign or malignant. A benign fluid-filled cyst may be drained using a fine needle, and no further treatment is needed. But if there is a solid tumour, it is more likely to be malignant, although it may also contain fluid cystic areas.

Alternatively, a laparotomy may be the first diagnostic procedure, or it may follow on directly after a laparoscopy. A laparotomy involves opening the abdomen to assess the problem. Any surgery then needed can also be carried out. This is a more major operation. The types of surgery which may be needed would be discussed with the woman beforehand. If you are in this situation, you must be sure you understand and agree with what may need to be done before you sign a consent form.

If a laparotomy follows a laparoscopy, you would be asked to give your formal consent to any surgery before you have the laparoscopy, as you wouldn't recover consciousness between the two procedures.

Could you explain the types of surgery which may be necessary?

What you have done will depend on whether you are of child-bearing age, and on whether the tumour is benign or malignant. The younger you are, and the less serious the condition, the less the surgeon will remove. Here we describe the treatments for benign tumours.

A benign cyst in a young woman will be 'shelled out' from the ovary and the ovary stitched back together, using soluble stitches which dissolve away.

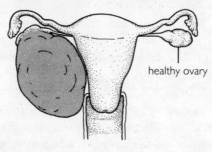

healthy ovary

A benign cyst which requires draining by syringe or 'shelling out' surgically, depending on its contents.

In an older woman who has completed her family, the whole ovary may be removed. This is quite a straightforward procedure called an oophorectomy. The ovary is attached to the womb by a ligament; this is simply cut, and the ovary freed from its supporting tissue on the side wall of the pelvis, and removed.

If the woman is past the menopause, the surgeon will probably remove the other healthy ovary to prevent the same problem recurring.

Where polycystic ovaries have not been cured by drug treatment, surgery will be carried out. There are two possible procedures. The traditional method is just to remove a wedge of tissue from each ovary during a laparotomy. This is now being replaced by laser treatment. A laser beam is directed at the ovaries using a laparoscope and used literally to drill holes in their surface. Laser laparoscopy is not a major procedure, like a laparotomy, and the woman can go home the following day. The after-effects of this procedure are no different to the normal minor effects following laparoscopy*. Why these treatments work is unknown, but breaking up the surface of the ovary does help the condition.

Tell me what to expect if I have a laparotomy to remove cysts.

You will be in hospital for about a week following a laparotomy and removal of benign cysts, or of an ovary. Read Chapter 2 on Preparing for Surgery before going into hospital.

This is what to expect after the operation.

1. You will have some abdominal soreness and discomfort, but it shouldn't be acute. Painkillers will be given if necessary. Sometimes the area is simply numb.
2. The anaesthetic may leave you feeling sick, but this shouldn't be severe, or last more than a few hours. In any event, drugs can be given by injection to relieve nausea.
3. There may be a drain* (a slim tube) from the incision to remove any collection of fluid following the operation. This is most likely if a cyst has ruptured, releasing fluid into the pelvic cavity. A drain is usually removed within about four days.
4. You may be on a drip* (a tube attached to a needle inserted into a vein in your hand or arm) to replace fluid lost during surgery and because you will not be able to drink straight after the operation. You will probably need this for about two days. If you need a blood transfusion*, this will be given the same way. It is unlikely that a catheter* will be necessary after this operation (a tube inserted in your urethra to help you urinate).
5. You will be out of bed within two days.
6. The stitches in the incision in your abdomen will be removed before you leave hospital. You will probably feel you have to walk carefully, and you may not be able to straighten up properly, but this is nothing to worry about. You will get over this as you heal.

After any major operation, it is often the shock to the system, rather than the operation itself, which hits you hardest, particularly when you first leave hospital.

How long do I need to recover fully?

You need to take things easy for about a month to allow for
internal healing. This means not doing anything which could
strain your abdominal muscles, such as driving the car or lifting
anything heavy; advice on this is given on page 111. You will
be advised not to have sexual intercourse until you have had
your post-operative hospital check after six weeks. Of course,
this doesn't mean that all sexual pleasuring has to cease before
then. You should be able to resume full normal life once you
have had your check-up.

What size is in the incision for a laparotomy? I'm worried about being left
with a large scar.

The usual incision is no more than about 10 cm (4 in) long
and is made across the lower abdomen on the pubic hairline.
However, for larger tumours the incision may go vertically up
the abdomen, its length being whatever is necessary for the surgeon to perform the operation safely. But the surgeon will make
every effort to keep the incision as small as possible. In any
case, the scar will eventually fade.

Supposing a malignant tumour is found; what is the treatment then?

This will require more extensive surgery. A hysterectomy to
remove the womb, Fallopian tubes and both ovaries will need
to be carried out. Chapter 15 on Hysterectomy gives information and advice on this major operation.

If malignancy is suspected, it is likely that the woman would
be asked to come into hospital about three days before the operation (rather than the usual day before). This is in case cancer has
become more widespread, involving the bowel, sections of which
may need to be removed. During the time prior to the operation,
she would be put on a fluid-only diet for two days and given laxatives to clear the bowel; some laxatives by mouth and some by
enema (a tube inserted into the anus through which liquid is
passed into the bowel to assist the clearance of solid waste).

Although this is not pleasant or dignified, it has considerable
benefits surgically. If sections of the bowel have to be removed
and it is well prepared before surgery, the surgeon would be
more likely to join the bowel together after taking out any cancerous parts, rather than performing a colostomy. But, however
well prepared the bowel is, a minority of women will still need
a colostomy.

Could you explain what a colostomy involves?

A colostomy involves diverting the bowel to an opening in the
abdomen, called a stoma, through which solid waste passes and
is collected in a lightweight bag; adhesive seals attach the bag to
the skin around the stoma. It is changed as necessary.

Of course, this is a major operation in itself, and can be a
severe blow to a woman's self-image and self-esteem. Being
admitted to hospital a few days before surgery thus also allows
time for counselling. A specialist stoma care nurse will give
advice on the use of the colostomy bag, and is experienced in
helping a patient come to terms with the operation both before
and after surgery. Recovery from this operation would simply
be part of recovery from having the hysterectomy. The stoma
care nurse would continue giving help and support during
home visits after the woman has left hospital.

Will the nurse be able to reassure me about living with a colostomy?

Yes, the nurse will be able to give reassurance that there is no
need to worry about odour, or about the bag showing through
your clothes. It won't come adrift either, nor interfere with a
woman's sex life, if she and her partner can adjust psychologically to this change. Counselling can help with any such problems and there are colostomy support groups; see the Useful
Addresses section. It is a fact that famous and glamorous stars
have had this operation and have successfully resumed their
lives.

Is a colostomy always permanent?

A colostomy is not necessarily permanent, and surgery to restore the bowel may be possible after about a year. This gives time for about six months of chemotherapy (treatment with anti-cancer drugs). Occasionally, radiotherapy may be used in addition to, or instead of, chemotherapy. (These treatments are explained in Chapter 17.) The patient's progress can then be assessed for another six months.

Questions Women Most Often Ask About Ovarian Tumours

Can all benign cysts be cured by surgery?

Yes, removal of the cysts – or of the affected ovary – is usually a complete cure. If functional cysts recur, this may be due to hormonal problems, which are treatable, or to stress, which can affect our hormones. Help with reducing stress is given in Chapter 18.

If I had to have an ovary removed, what effect would this have?

It wouldn't have any noticeable effect. If you are of childbearing age, the remaining ovary would continue to produce enough hormones to support fertility, although the chances of conception would be slightly reduced. You would not experience menopausal symptoms*, as these are due to diminished levels of the hormone oestrogen secreted by the ovaries; the remaining ovary would compensate.

Would I have menopausal symptoms if both my ovaries had to be removed?

If you have not yet gone through the menopause it is very unlikely that both your ovaries would have to be removed to cure benign cysts. As already described, both ovaries are removed either when the woman is past the menopause or where there is a malignant tumour. Ovarian cancer is more common in older, post-menopausal women, who are not affected by menopausal symptoms after surgery.

In a younger woman who has had both ovaries removed, hormone replacement therapy (HRT) can replace the missing oestrogen and relieve menopausal symptoms. But HRT cannot be given if cancer has spread from the breast, as sometimes happens (i.e. the ovarian tumour is a 'secondary', the 'primary' tumour being in the breast). Oestrogen encourages the spread of breast cancer*. A woman who has had ovarian cancer and who has a strong family history of breast cancer may also be advised not to have HRT.

Information about HRT and self-help with menopausal symptoms is given on pages 213–16.

Am I likely to get ovarian cancer?

Although it is not a common cancer, it does affect more women than other cancers of the reproductive organs, which is why regular check-ups are so vital, particularly if you could be at risk.

How would I know if I were at risk of getting this cancer?

There are factors which seem to put certain women more at risk:

- having a family history of the disease (one or more of their female relatives have had ovarian cancer)
- being childless
- having had breast cancer

Are there any ways of reducing the risk of ovarian cancer?

There are two ways which may help, even though they appear contradictory. One is to have a large family, the other is to take the combined oral contraceptive pill. There is in fact no contradiction here, because both the pill and pregnancy prevent ovulation. Why this should be helpful isn't clear, but research has shown that it apparently does have a protective effect.

Is there any other way of detecting early ovarian cancer in addition to routine check-ups?

Yes. A very early sign is an increased blood-flow in the ovaries. This can be detected by colour ultrasound*, which is available in some hospitals to women who could be at risk. It is very well worth enquiring about this if any of the risk factors mentioned are relevant to you.

What are the chances of a cure after treatment for ovarian cancer?

If it is caught early, the chances are good. Unfortunately, in many cases ovarian cancer has spread beyond the pelvis by the time the diagnosis is made, making the outlook not so good. Even so, with a combination of skilled surgery, radiotherapy and chemotherapy, many women do extremely well.

13

CERVICAL CANCER AND PRE-CANCER

No woman need have cervical cancer. It is entirely avoidable if the right steps are taken. Having a cervical smear test regularly is vital, because this quick and easy test detects early changes to the cervix which could lead to cancer.

The cervix is the round pad of flesh which protrudes into the top of the vagina – it can be felt with your finger – and is the entrance to the womb. It is usually called the 'neck of the womb'. If there are any changes to the cervix, they can be completely cured by simple procedures which can include surgery, and there is no reason to fear any of this. Here we give the essential facts which every woman should know about the disease, and the treatments required. Just as important, we also aim to show how you can help yourself by making the right decisions about your health.

We hear so much about cervical cancer these days. Does this mean I'm likely to get it?

It's not one of the more common kinds of cancer, even though it is one of the most emotive health issues of our time. This is because it is linked to sexual intercourse and the more liberated lifestyles of both sexes today. It is on the increase, but promiscuity is not necessarily a factor. You could be at risk whether you've had only one partner, or more. This does not necessarily mean that you are likely to get cervical cancer. It simply means that all women who have ever been sexually active need to be aware that there is a risk, and should know how to protect themselves. Questions about the possible causes of cervical cancer – and why sexual behaviour is a factor – are answered later in this chapter (see pages 188–90).

How can I tell if I've got cervical cancer?

The biggest problem with cervical cancer is that there are usually no early warning signs that the disease is developing. In most cases the woman feels perfectly fit. This is why it is so vital to have regular smear tests even when you have no reason to think anything is wrong. Unfortunately, symptoms generally occur only when cancer has spread from the cervix into the womb (uterus) and pelvis, and possibly also the vagina. There can then be deep pain in the pelvic area and during sex, bleeding after intercourse, between periods or even after the menopause. There may occasionally be an offensive-smelling discharge. Although there can be other, less serious causes of such symptoms, a medical check-up is essential if you have any of these problems.

What happens if you develop cervical cancer?

If the disease is allowed to develop, the surgery then necessary can sadly result in sterility for life, which means, of course, you cannot have children. This is particularly tragic for younger women who may not have started families.

The more advanced the disease becomes, the more difficult it is to cure. **But all this is easily prevented**.

How can I be sure I'm not developing cervical cancer?

By having cervical smear tests as often as your doctor advises. Many of the women who develop cervical cancer have never had a smear test, or have neglected to continue having the test after being given one normal result. As we have already said, the smear test is quick and easy to carry out, and it detects early abnormal changes at a stage when they can be cured by simple procedures; these procedures do not affect a woman 's ability to have a baby. Self-help methods of preventing cervical cancer are given later in this chapter (see pages 188–9).

Does the smear test hurt?

Not at all. A lubricated speculum is inserted into the vagina to open it so the cervix can be seen. The speculum may feel a bit cold, and if you are tense it may be uncomfortable, so try to relax: taking some deep breaths and breathing out slowly may help. The smear test itself involves the doctor or nurse simply removing some surface cells from your cervix using a wooden spatula or a special brush. This may be mildly uncomfortable, but some women hardly feel a thing, and it takes only a few seconds.

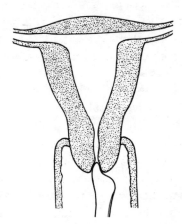

The smear test: cells being removed from the cervix by spatula for examination.

Will anything else be done if I have a smear test?

You may well have a pelvic examination*, but this depends on whether the smear is taken by a doctor or nurse. A doctor may give you this general check, because a smear test provides the ideal opportunity for it.

I feel rather embarrassed at the thought of having a pelvic examination* or cervical smear test, and this puts me off going to the doctor.

Quite a lot of women feel like this, sometimes because the doctor is a man. Remember that doctors are professionals, and that they regard what they are doing as just part of their job. Many will do their best to put you at ease. There is more on coping with the 'embarrassment factor' in Chapter 1. Where the smear test is concerned, remember that it could save your life.

How will I be told the result of the smear test?

The cells which have been removed are sent for analysis; you will either receive the result by post or be given it personally by your doctor.

I know I should have regular smear tests, but I dread finding out 'the worst'.

Unfortunately, people are inclined to put off doing the sensible thing if they have fears about it. But the vast majority of smear test results are in fact 'negative', which means nothing is wrong. If you do have a 'positive' result, it certainly does not always mean you have cancer – this is true of most 'positive' smears.

What should I do if I have a 'positive' smear?

First of all, don't panic. See your doctor as soon as possible. S/he may contact you personally with the result anyway. Find out what the result means. Reading the next question will help you with this. Above all, don't just assume you have cancer.

Could you explain what a 'positive' smear means?

If you have a 'positive' result, you will very likely hear your doctor using the medical terms listed overleaf. It will help you, and save time, if you already know them. It will also be easier to understand the treatment proposed if you have a clear idea of why it is needed.

A 'positive' result can mean one of the following.

1. There are mild abnormal changes to your cervical cells. Three medical terms are used to describe these slight changes, but in essence they all refer to the same thing. They are mild dyskaryosis, mild dysplasia, and CIN 1.
2. There are moderate changes to the cells; this is known as moderate dyskaryosis, moderate dysplasia, or CIN 2. This means that the cells are continuing to change and show more abnormalities.
3. There are further abnormal changes to the cells, called severe dyskaryosis, severe dysplasia, or CIN 3. These are sometimes also referred to as carcinoma-in-situ, although some doctors don't use the term because it sounds so frightening. But if you hear these words, there's no need to think you have cancer. The term means that even though many of the cells show severe changes, these cells are still only on the surface of your cervix.

None of the changes just described are in fact cancer. They are called pre-cancerous changes because they could develop into cancer.

I don't understand the difference between pre-cancer and cervical cancer.

Cervical cancer exists only when cancerous cells have broken through the membrane − called the basement membrane − which separates the surface cells of the cervix from its deeper tissues (see illustration on page 178).

Can all pre-cancerous changes be cured?

In most cases they are curable. The abnormal surface cells can be removed well before they spread any deeper, and this treatment can be repeated if necessary. Sometimes, however, mild abnormal changes can cure themselves without treatment − the cells simply revert to normal. This cannot be relied upon to happen, and so if smears repeatedly show mild changes, further tests will be carried out. Moderate and severe changes will always be investigated further.

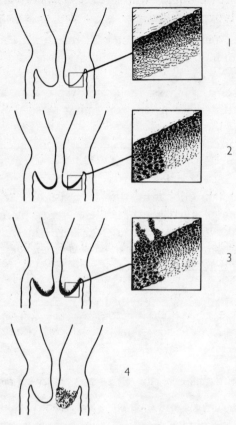

The contrast between (1) normal cells on the cervix and (2) severe pre-cancerous changes, which can be completely cured. (3) Micro-invasion is the earliest stage of cervical cancer: abnormal cells have penetrated the basement membrane separating surface cells from the deeper tissues. (4) Actual cancer present as a growth on the cervix.

How are further tests carried out after a 'positive' smear?

These usually take place in the out-patient clinic of a hospital. You will be given an examination using an instrument called a colposcope – the examination is called colposcopy. This involves lying on a couch with your legs supported comfortably apart by stirrups. As with the smear test, your vagina is opened with a speculum. The cervix is then wiped with acetic acid (dilute vinegar), which is usually painless but may sting slightly, or with iodine. These liquids will reveal any abnormal areas. You will have a brownish discharge for a day or so afterwards if iodine is used, but this is nothing to worry about.

The colposcope – which is like a binocular telescope – is positioned about 15 cm (6 in) from the vulva (the vaginal area) to make a good view of the cervix possible. The doctor examines the cervix through it; this takes about five minutes. A photograph may be taken of your cervix for future reference. Further samples of cells will also be removed, as well as a small piece of solid tissue from an abnormal area for detailed analysis. This is called a biopsy. It may hurt momentarily, although some women don't feel a thing. A tampon may be inserted afterwards, as there can be a little bleeding.

Again, some women can feel embarrassed and nervous, even frightened, about this examination and the necessary tests. Try to relax – deep breathing may help – and don 't even consider what the doctor may be thinking about you. S/he will be concentrating on the examination, and may well explain what is happening as it goes along, to reassure you and so you know what to expect. The tests will tell the doctor which treatments are necessary. It will take a few days for the results to come through.

What will be done if I have to be treated for pre-cancer?

There are several procedures for the treatment of pre-cancerous changes; they work to destroy all abnormal cells. The treatment given depends on how mild or severe the changes are. But all treatments are quite straightforward, so you need have no fears about will be done. Below is a description of the different treatments. Some of them can be given in the out-patient clinic of a hospital, allowing you to go home directly afterwards.

LASER TREATMENT
Laser treatment is usually done under local anaesthetic at an outpatient clinic. The anaesthetic is injected into the cervix with a

very fine dental needle, so it hurts less than other routine injections. Abnormal cells are then heated so fast, using a powerful beam of laser light, that they simply evaporate. You won't feel a thing while this is happening. All stages of pre-cancer can be treated this way. Treatment can take about fifteen minutes. The cervix will heal well.

ELECTRODIATHERMY
This procedure also uses heat, but in this case the heat comes from an electrode placed on the cervix. Treatment is carried out under general anaesthetic in hospital, so you will probably be in hospital overnight. It, too, can be used to treat all stages of pre-cancer.

HOT WIRE CAUTERY
This is similar to electrodiathermy. Healing is good with both treatments.

DIATHERMY LOOP
Diathermy loop is a more recent treatment which acts to remove the affected part of the cervix using a low-voltage wire loop. It takes only five to ten seconds and is done under local anaesthetic at an out-patient clinic. All stages of pre-cancer can be treated. Because a whole piece of tissue is removed which can be sent for laboratory analysis, this technique can be both a diagnosis and a treatment. It may be used in place of methods which simply destroy abnormal tissue.

COLD COAGULATION
Contrary to its name, cold coagulation is also a heat treatment, although the heat applied is much lower in temperature than for the other treatments. No anaesthetic is required. It may cause a mild period-like pain and, if so, you will be given painkillers. It takes only a few minutes at an out-patient clinic. This treatment is used for mild or moderate pre-cancerous changes.

CRYOTHERAPY
Cryotherapy destroys abnormal cells by freezing them. No anaesthetic is needed but, as with cold coagulation, you feel a

mild period-like pain which can be relieved with painkillers. Treatment takes about 10 or 15 minutes at an out-patient clinic. Cryotherapy is more likely to be used for treating mild or moderate changes.

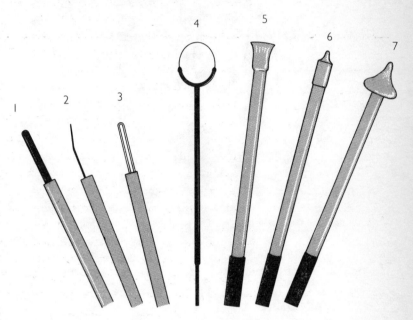

Some instruments used to treat cervical pre-cancer: (1) and (2) electrodiathermy; (3) hot wire cautery; (4) diathermy loop; (5) and (6) cold coagulation; (7) cryotherapy.

CONE BIOPSY

This can be both a test and a treatment. It is a type of surgery carried out only when the doctor is not satisfied that the usual tests have shown all the abnormal areas on the cervix. What happens then is that the centre of the cervix is removed in a section resembling a cone or cylinder in shape. This larger piece can then be examined in detail. A cone biopsy may be done under general anaesthetic, which means a stay of a few days in hospital. But it can sometimes be carried out using a laser under local anaesthetic, so treatment can be given at an out-patient clinic and you can go home the same day.

Usually the result is that all abnormal cells have been

removed. But if there are signs that they go deeper into the cervix, further treatment will depend on how far they have spread (see page 185).

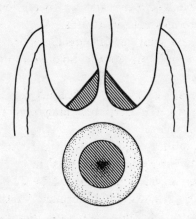

Cone biopsy removes a cone- or cylinder-shaped piece of tissue from the centre of the cervix for examination. Used to determine the extent of abnormal changes, it can be both an aid to diagnosis and a treatment.

None of these treatments will prevent you from having a baby.

HYSTERECTOMY*

Hysterectomy* (removal of the womb) is not often used to treat pre-cancer. But sometimes there may be signs of on-going abnormalities in spite of repeated treatments; pre-cancer may extend up the cervical canal to the womb, out of reach from below, making a hysterectomy necessary.

I will be having out-patient treatment for pre-cancer. What preparations do I need to make, and how will I feel afterwards?

Here are the main things to bear in mind.

1. Make sure you are not about to have a period. This can make any bleeding from the cervix worse, since the area is about to start bleeding anyway. Don't be in the middle of a period, either.

2. Be sure you understand exactly what will be done. This will help you feel much less anxious.

3. Wear clothes which can be removed easily below the waist before treatment, and which are loose, as this will be more comfortable afterwards.

4. Take a friend with you, if possible – or, better still, your partner – who can literally hold your hand throughout treatment.

5. Try to relax, as this will reduce any discomfort and help you to feel calm. Deep breathing may help, as already suggested.

6. Be prepared for bleeding afterwards, or a watery discharge which may have dark 'bits' in it. This can last several weeks, so don't be surprised by it. If it worries you do contact your doctor or hospital. Sanitary towels need to be worn, because tampons increase the risk of infection.

7 Antiseptic cream may be applied to your cervix after treatment, and for a while you may need to insert it into your vagina (using a special applicator) to help the healing process. You may also be asked to take antibiotics to prevent infection and help healing.

8. Some women feel more 'socked' by treatment than they expected. You may feel weepy and low afterwards. It will be a great help if someone sympathetic can be with you. Take things easy, too. For instance, don't plan to go out that evening, and get some early nights. On the other hand, many women feel only relief that their condition has been cured.

I am going into hospital to be treated for pre-cancer under a general anaesthetic. I need some advice on what will happen.

You will be in the hands of professionals, and this alone is a reassuring thought. Read Chapter 2 on Preparing for Surgery: it offers detailed guidance for in-patients, but here is some advice specific to treatment for pre-cancer.

1. As with out-patient treatment for pre-cancer, make sure you will not be having a period at the time you are having treatment.

2. When you come round from the anaesthetic after treatment, you will feel a dull ache in your abdomen. You will be wearing a sanitary towel. If you have had a cone biopsy, you may have a cramping, period-like pain and be rather uncomfortable – this will be due to the gauze dressing inside your vagina. It is there is to stop the bleeding and is packed in quite tightly. A catheter (a tube) inserted in your urethra enables you to pass urine. The dressing (and the catheter) will usually be removed the day after surgery; this can also be uncomfortable. Painkillers will always be given, should you need them at any time.

3. A general anaesthetic can make you feel drowsy and sick, so you will probably stay in hospital for up to 48 hours.

4. You may be given antibiotics to take which will help healing and prevent infection. Again – as after out-patient treatment – don't be surprised if you bleed or have a discharge for some weeks. This is normal. Wear sanitary towels, not tampons, to avoid infection. And if you have any worries do contact the hospital or your doctor.

5. Occasionally there is some quite heavy bleeding 7 to 14 days after treatment, especially following a cone biopsy, and this usually means infection is present. Contact your doctor straight away, as you may need to be re-admitted to hospital. Treatment may be by packing the vagina with gauze to stop the bleeding from the cervix; this is inserted under a light general anaesthetic. The gauze will remain inside for 48 hours, during which time you will need a catheter in the bladder to pass urine, and you will be on antibiotics. Removal of any dressing may be uncomfortable, but you can have painkillers if necessary. Usually you will leave hospital the same day.

6. After a cone biopsy, you may notice what some women have described as 'small threadlike worms' appearing from your vagina during healing. These are simply bits of

the soluble stitches in your cervix which are dissolving, and are nothing to worry about.

7. It usually takes a little longer to recover from in-patient treatment than if you have been an out-patient. So plan to have a quiet few days. It will help if you can have someone with you to whom you can really talk. You may feel depressed and be glad of a shoulder to cry on, although this isn't true of all women. Some recover quite speedily, with few emotional after-effects.

How long does it take the cervix to heal after treatment for pre-cancer?

Usually a minimum of two weeks, but it may take up to five weeks if you've had a cone biopsy. It is inadvisable to take vigorous exercise or to have sex before then, but these will also depend on your doctor's advice and on how you feel. Physical and emotional closeness to a partner is often especially important at this time, so lovemaking without penetration can be very supportive and reassuring. But if there are problems in the relationship, perhaps as a result of your having had pre-cancer, it may help you to read the questions at the end of this chapter.

I've had treatment for pre-cancer, and want to know if there will be any long-term effects.

There are usually none. Occasionally a cone biopsy causes painful periods if the entrance to the cervix tightens, but this can be put right. A cone biopsy may also increase the risk of a miscarriage* in pregnancy; this can be prevented by inserting the 'purse-string' stitch described on page 136.

You have said that if abnormal cells have spread into the cervix, treatment depends on how far they go. What does this mean?

It means that cervical cancer is present. If it is caught at an early stage when the spread is very limited (this is called micro-invasion − see illustration on page 178), it may be possible to remove all the cancerous cells using a cone biopsy. Regular checks for cancer will then be needed, and treatment can be repeated if necessary. So, if you are young and want children, this treatment may be carried out because you can still have a baby afterwards. In other circumstances, a hysterectomy* is likely to be advised, but this is something your gynaecologist will discuss with you in relation to your particular needs. If cancer appears to go deeper, tests will be done to find out how far it has spread.

How do they find out how far cervical cancer has spread?

The womb lining can be removed by D & C (dilation and curettage)* for examination. A D & C is often done during a cone biopsy anyway, in order to determine the spread within the cervix. Various tests can show how far cancer has spread outside the cervix. An ultrasound scan* or CT scan* will show what is happening in the pelvis.

A CT scan uses X-rays* to record cross-sectional 'slices' of the body, which are collected by computer to produce complete pictures on a video screen. All tissues and organs in the pelvis can be seen, including the lymph nodes. The lymph nodes are vital to our natural defence against disease, known as the 'immune system', so if cancer cells have taken them over, the disease can spread more easily, causing tumours in other parts of the body.

A lymphangiogram shows specifically whether or not the lymph nodes have been invaded. It involves injecting harmless dye into the feet which then travels to the pelvis where it can be seen on an X-ray. Harmless dye can also be injected into a vein in the arm; this travels to the kidneys so they show up on an X-ray; this is called an intravenous urogram (IVU). We must stress that such tests are needed by only a minority of women.

Could you explain more about the lymph nodes?

The lymph nodes are located in many parts of the body, including the pelvis, armpits, chest and neck. Their function is to filter a clear fluid called lymph, which is derived from the blood. The tissues are bathed in lymph as it travels round the body via the lymphatic system before returning to the bloodstream.

The nodes act rather like sieves to prevent impurities (such as cancer cells and other diseases or infections) from entering the lymphatic system and the bloodstream. The nodes also produce a type of white blood cell called a lymphocyte. These cells help the immune system to demolish the invading enemies. As already mentioned, if the lymph nodes have lost the battle against cancer cells, the disease can spread to other parts of the body. A sign of the lymph nodes acting against invaders of all kinds is when they swell and harden.

If I find I have cervical cancer, what is the treatment?

Treatment is never just routine; it is planned to suit each woman, so your gynaecologist would discuss this with you. However, treatment is likely to involve hysterectomy* and/or radiotherapy*. The type of hysterectomy will, again, depend on how far the cancer has spread. Some hysterectomies involve removing not only the womb and cervix, but also tissue around the cervix, plus the lymph nodes in the pelvis.

Radiotherapy means that the diseased area is bombarded with X-rays, which destroy cancer cells. This can be carried out before and after surgery, or if surgery is not possible because cancer is too widespread. Chapter 15 gives details of the different types of operation and the radiotherapy needed for cancer – and how to cope with treatment.

Much can be done to treat cervical cancer, but these are major treatments and you will very probably need a lot of emotional support. If you have a partner and are physically and emotionally close to him, this will be a great help. Sometimes the experience of cervical cancer and pre-cancer brings a couple closer – although, sadly, this is not always the case. As we have already said, if you have relationship problems, the questions at the end of this chapter may help. And, of course, there are other sources of support; see pages 190–1.

I've heard that there are new 'miracle' drugs which can cure cervical cancer. Is this true?

It's still too early to be absolutely certain about this. It is true that trials involving a powerful 'cocktail' of drugs have shown encouraging results in some women who have not been cured by surgery or radiotherapy. The drugs are given as a course of injections. They can have debilitating side-effects during treatment; these may include nausea and temporary hair loss. But the good news is that cancer does seem to have been completely cured in some of the women treated. It is hoped that drug treatment will eventually replace surgery and radiotherapy, but this stage is at present still some way off.

Questions Women Most Often Ask About Cervical Cancer and Pre-cancer

What causes cervical cancer?

Like other cancers, cervical cancer happens when normal cell functioning goes wrong. Cells normally divide to make new ones which replace old ones that die, and this renewal happens throughout our lives. Cells which go on dividing uncontrollably form a growth or tumour, and if this tumour spreads to other parts of the body it is said to be cancerous or malignant (benign growths do not spread beyond themselves). What starts this process in cervical cancer isn't known for certain. The genital herpes virus, which is sexually transmitted, used to be a prime suspect, but it now seems more likely that certain strains of the genital wart virus, also transmitted during intercourse, are to blame. What initiates the change is unclear, but it would seems to be more common in women who smoke. Starting sex when very young also appears to be a factor, but this may be because the cervix is more vulnerable in the early years after puberty.

How can I protect myself from cervical cancer?

1. By having regular smear tests at the intervals recommended by your doctor, as already advised.

2. By always using barrier contraception in any non-established relationship. The condom and, to a lesser extent, the diaphragm and cervical cap provide protection from the wart virus and also other sexually transmitted diseases. Anti-HIV/AIDS campaigns have promoted the use of condoms, and hopefully this will help prevent cervical cancer and pre-cancer as well. HIV attacks the body's immune system (see below), so condoms are vital. Some doctors, particularly in the USA, recommend that barrier contraception always be used after a 'positive' smear, but this has to be a personal decision, and will of course depend on such factors as whether children are wanted.

3. By adopting a healthier lifestyle. Anything which reduces immunity (the body's natural defence against disease) can make cervical cancer and pre-cancer more liable to develop if the woman has been at risk. Such things include stress, poor diet, lack of exercise and, above all, smoking. Chapter 18 includes advice on healthy living.

What will happen if a woman is pregnant when she has a 'positive' smear?

This is a difficult but fortunately uncommon situation. A woman's immunity is naturally reduced by pregnancy, making it more likely that any abnormal changes to the cervix will develop faster. Giving treatment at this time, however, is avoided if possible, as it may mean that the pregnancy cannot continue. The decision will depend on the severity of the condition and on the woman's feelings. On the other hand, nine months is not a long time to wait, so a woman may be advised to have the baby and then be treated immediately thereafter.

I've had a 'positive' smear and am afraid to say anything in case people think I'm promiscuous. In fact, I've only had two sex partners and am now in a long-term faithful relationship with one of them, so this can't be true, can it?

The view that any woman who has a 'positive' smear − or who is unfortunate enough to develop cervical cancer − must have a different man every night of the week causes much unnecessary guilt and anxiety. As said at the start of the chapter, you don't have to be promiscuous to be at risk – and it is false to assume that it is always the woman's fault. At the same time, there is evidence that the risks increase with the number of sexual partners – whether it is the man or the woman who has them. A woman in a relationship where neither partner has had sex with anyone else is therefore at no risk. But fewer people today have had only one partner in the whole of their lives. So if you, or your partner, have ever had sex with anyone else, you can be at risk.

I have such hostile feelings towards my partner after having treatment for pre-cancer. I know he's had previous partners and I think he's been unfaithful to me and that this caused the problem. Am I right to be suspicious?

Such feelings are far from unusual and, as said above, they can stem from social attitudes which attach guilt and blame to the disease – and men are being blamed more often now. The genital wart virus (thought to be the main culprit) can be present without symptoms in both men and women. It can be transmitted from one partner to the other long after the original infection occurred with a previous partner. Even if visible warts on the genitals have been treated, this doesn't always eradicate the virus. So your problem doesn't necessarily mean he has been unfaithful to you. But pre-cancer can become the focus for hurt and resentment about a partner's sexual past or his present behaviour.

My partner just doesn't understand how I feel about having pre-cancer, and my relationship is on the rocks due to his lack of sympathy. What can I do?

Problems which may already exist in a relationship, such as lack of sympathy and communication, can be made worse by the shock and stress of having pre-cancer. Or it may be that he doesn't know how to handle his feelings about your problem. Whatever the reason, it is always worth seeking professional counselling help, either on your own or with your partner if possible. There are also support groups and telephone help-lines specially for women with health and relationship problems. Your doctor or hospital will tell you where to find help locally; see also the Useful Addresses section at the end of this book.

I no longer have a partner, and I don't want to have sex again after what has happened to me with pre-cancer. It doesn't seem worth the risk and the hurt, does it?

This is a decision some women make. Cervical problems are bound to influence your sexual feelings strongly. But it could be worth talking out your feelings with a counsellor. Having a condition of the cervix doesn't mean that you can never have a rewarding sexual relationship.

I'm being treated for cervical cancer. Is there anything I can do to help myself fight the disease?

Yes, you can build your physical and psychological strength through healthier living (see Chapter 18). Counselling and simply talking to other women who have had the disease can also be immensely helpful. If a hysterectomy and/or radiotherapy has caused problems in a sexual relationship, counselling can be very worthwhile. See Chapter 15.

You are likely to find that other people who are being treated for cancer at the same hospital or clinic can be most kind and supportive. You too may discover strengths in yourself which enable you to help them. Above all, you can be sure of one thing: you do not have to be alone with your problem.

14

CANCER OF THE WOMB

The possibility of having any of the cancers is extremely alarming, but − fortunately − if caught early cancer of the womb is one of the more curable. There are advance warning symptoms (as is not the case with cervical cancer*), and it is vital that you know what these symptoms are. If you experience any of them, however, it doesn't necessarily mean you have this disease (which is also called uterine or endometrial cancer). Other benign causes are in fact much more likely. Even so, you must have a check-up right away. Here we give essential information about the disease, to reassure any woman facing diagnosis or treatment that she can have an excellent chance of recovery after surgery.

What are the early symptoms of cancer of the womb?

Before the menopause, the first symptoms may be prolonged periods, or bleeding between periods − or a combination of both. After the menopause, vaginal bleeding or a blood-stained (reddish-brown) discharge are the usual symptoms. Occasionally, a constant pale yellow discharge may be a symptom after the menopause. Bleeding after intercourse also needs to be reported to your doctor promptly. We must again stress that these symptoms do not inevitably indicate cancer of the womb (uterus). Heavy irregular bleeding can result from a hormonal imbalance*, which may respond to hormone treatment, or may be caused by fibroids* or polyps* − benign growths which can be surgically removed. Polyps can also be the cause of bleeding after intercourse.

How common is cancer of the womb?

It is less common than either cancer of the ovaries* or of the cervix*. It differs considerably from cervical cancer, which is associated with a virus infection and rarely, if ever, occurs in women who have never been sexually active. Cancer of the womb is more likely to affect women who have not had children (i.e. women with fertility problems – see below) and those who are very overweight; the majority of women affected are also past the menopause.

What causes the disease?

Almost certainly it is linked to the ovarian hormone oestrogen. This is secreted by the ovaries, and in the first half of the menstrual cycle following a period it causes the endometrium (the womb lining) to grow and thicken. Ovulation – the release of a ripe egg from one of the ovaries – usually occurs in the middle of the cycle, and a second ovarian hormone, progesterone, then 'balances' the effects of oestrogen by preparing the endometrium for its function: to receive a fertilized egg and start a pregnancy. But if the woman fails to ovulate (produce a ripe egg), then there is little or no progesterone and the endometrium will grow but not function. Excessive oestrogen which is 'unopposed' by progesterone may eventually result in unrestricted growth of the endometrium, and this is cancer.

Why would a woman have this hormone imbalance?

As just mentioned, if a woman fails to ovulate she will produce oestrogen but little or no progesterone. Failure to ovulate is a common cause of infertility; this is why uterine cancer is linked to women who have not had children (but who have not been practising abstinence from sex or contraception). Lack of ovulation may have no obvious cause, or it can be due to an imbalance in the hormones which control ovulation, and this can be treated with drugs. Other causes can be a disorder called polycystic ovaries*, or simply stress. But the woman herself cannot know whether or not she is ovulating.

Also, body fat produces oestrogen quite independently, so very overweight women will tend to produce more oestrogen than women who are slim. This oestrogen will also be 'unopposed' by progesterone, hence the link between uterine cancer and obesity.

Hormone replacement therapy (HRT)*, which is given to relieve menopausal symptoms*, used to be suspect because originally only oestrogen was replaced, but now this is balanced by taking progestogen (synthetic progesterone); HRT is therefore no longer considered a risk.

Are there any other risk factors?

No, but there are associated factors which can affect women who have the risk factors already mentioned. These associated factors are:

- high blood-pressure
- diabetes
- fibroids

Women affected by any of these associated factors should therefore be alert to any early symptoms which could indicate cancer of the womb. But if any of these factors affect you, it doesn't mean that you are inevitably going to develop the disease; they can also be present without there being this danger.

Will a cervical smear test done during a routine check-up show cancer of the womb?*

Occasionally it does, but it cannot be relied upon to diagnose cancer of the womb. The smear test removes cells from the entrance to the womb (the cervix), not from inside the womb.

This is why any of the symptoms described earlier must be reported to your doctor without delay.

How is cancer of the womb diagnosed?

By D & C (dilation and curettage)*, which is a simple surgical method of removing samples of womb lining (a biopsy) for analysis under a microscope. The procedure requires at most an overnight stay in hospital and can often be performed on a day-patient basis. You will receive the results from the hospital or your own doctor. But, as already stated, if you are having a D & C for the symptoms described, it doesn't necessarily mean you have cancer.

Does this cancer spread in stages?

Yes. It is slow-growing, and early diagnosis may simply show changes to the endometrium (called hyperplasia), which may be considered a forerunner of cancer, i.e. the changes are pre-cancerous. In its early stages, cancer will only have invaded the inner wall of the womb – the muscle layer, or myometrium.

As time goes by the cancer will penetrate deeper into the muscle, until eventually it will spread to the Fallopian tubes, ovaries and around the pelvis. Only in exceptional cases will it spread around the body and affect other organs.

What are the treatments?

Hyperplasia may be treated by taking progestogen tablets, since these counteract the effects of oestrogen. The womb lining may return to normal; regular checks (biopsies) are needed thereafter. But if hyperplasia is severe or progestogen (synthetic progesterone) treatment ineffective, a hysterectomy (removal of the womb) is carried out.

If actual cancer is present in the womb lining, hysterectomy is the choice of treatment, and the womb is removed along with the Fallopian tubes and ovaries.

Depending on how far the cancer has spread, radiotherapy

may be given either before or (more commonly) after surgery. Sometimes chemotherapy (administering anti-cancer drugs) is used, often in the form of high doses of progestogen. But if the cancer is widespread, surgery and radiotherapy may not be possible; treatment with high doses of progestogen alone can do much to counteract its spread and reduce tumours, giving the woman a considerably increased life expectancy.

Read Chapter 15 on Hysterectomy and Chapter 17 on Radiotherapy and Chemotherapy for advice and reassurance on treatment. Fighting cancer is one of the greatest challenges anyone could face. There is much that can be done medically, and there are sources of emotional help and support available; these include counselling, self-help groups and telephone help-lines run by cancer charities.

Questions Women Most Often Ask About Cancer of the Womb

How would I know if I had advanced cancer?

As the disease progresses, there may be feelings of pressure and distention in the pelvis, severe cramping pains and the need to urinate frequently. Vaginal bleeding may become increasingly frequent and heavy. But as there are early warning symptoms, and this cancer takes time to develop, it can be treated long before it becomes this serious. Because it tends to occur during and after the menopause, a woman may delay seeing her doctor because she assumes that the symptoms are 'just something to do with natural changes at my time of life'. Never take that risk.

Is there anything I can do to protect myself from this cancer?

You can maintain your general health by adopting a sensible lifestyle (see Chapter 18 for advice) and by having regular medical checks. If you are very overweight, losing weight is certainly advisable. There is, however, no infallible way of preventing the changes which precede cancer of the womb. The most important thing you can do, therefore, to protect yourself is to be alert to any early symptoms and report them to your doctor promptly.

If this is one of the more curable cancers, what would be my chances of recovery?

Your chances after early diagnosis would be very good; when caught early around 90 per cent of women are successfully treated by surgery.

15

HYSTERECTOMY

Hysterectomy means removal of the womb. For many women, the term remains surrounded by myths and misinformation. A woman facing a hysterectomy can feel shocked and afraid, but the more she understands about it, and the more emotional support she has, the better she will be able to cope positively with this major operation and make a quick recovery afterwards. This is why it is so important to have full and sympathetic discussions about it beforehand.

There are in fact different types of hysterectomy, depending on the problems it is used to resolve. It is very helpful to know which type is being proposed and what is involved. In this chapter we will explain the operations, dispel the myths, and give you advice on recovery.

Will having a hysterectomy make me less female?

Absolutely not; this is just a myth. But this isn't to dismiss the greatest worry women often have about hysterectomy. The womb (or uterus) is a powerful symbol of femininity. It produces periods, which are a sign of female maturity; it make fulfilment as a mother possible; it is part of women's sexuality. Without it, a woman can feel a strong sense of loss – that she is somehow incomplete – especially if she is of childbearing age; the loss can be particularly great if she has not had the children she wants. Even women who do not want children, or who have all the children they want and may be past childbearing age, can still value it highly.

Not all women have these feelings, but many do have difficulty coming to terms with removal of the womb. Being without a womb does not make you any less female, however. You are female before you menstruate and are able to have children, and you remain a woman after the menopause when periods and fertility cease. Having a womb is certainly not essential to femininity.

Isn't hysterectomy more an operation for older women?

Some of the more common problems it is used to cure tend to need treatment when the woman is older, such as fibroids* or a prolapsed womb*. But problems such as endometriosis* and pelvic inflammatory disease (PID)*, which can cause severe pelvic pain, sometimes necessitate a hysterectomy at an earlier age.

How likely am I to have a hysterectomy?

It is certainly one of the more common gynaecological operations, although hysterectomies are performed more in some countries than others. The gynaecologist's attitude can also be a factor. A hysterectomy should be viewed as a treatment of last resort, to be used only when other treatments have proved ineffective, are not the best answer, or are not possible. A woman who is recommended to have a hysterectomy should always ask for a second opinion if she is in any doubt.

Fortunately, the number of hysterectomies is likely to be much reduced by more recent minor surgical procedures, called endometrial ablation* and endometrial resection*. These are used to treat heavy, painful, irregular periods, which have no obvious cause and have not responded to hormone treatment. These problems have been a prime reason for hysterectomies until now. But with these new treatments, the womb lining can be permanently removed so that periods cease, or are only very slight. They require a relatively light anaesthetic and only an overnight stay in hospital, or may even be performed on an out-patient basis under local anaesthetic, so the woman can go home the same day. Normal life can be resumed a few days afterwards. It is certainly worth enquiring about having one of these procedures if you suffer from severe menstrual problems which cannot be resolved.

I keep being told that hysterectomy will make a 'new woman' of me. Is this really true?

This is one of those comforting clichés which really can be true. If you have suffered debilitating, long-term symptoms, a hysterectomy can come as a relief and give you a new lease on life. For a woman who has cancer, it can be a life-saving procedure. A woman's awareness that a hysterectomy is being done for a good reason, and can bring a much-needed cure, is very important in helping her through the hospital experience, and with her recovery.

Is cancer a major reason for having a hysterectomy?

No. Although cancer is the greatest fear associated with hysterectomy, the majority of hysterectomies are carried out for other reasons.

What are the different types of hysterectomy, and why are they needed?

The problems for which hysterectomy can be needed are fully covered earlier in this book. Here we describe the operations, referring you to the relevant chapters for information on the problems, and on the alternative treatments to hysterectomy which may be possible.

VAGINAL HYSTERECTOMY

Vaginal hysterectomy is the only operation which removes the womb and cervix (neck of the womb) via the vagina. It is widely know as the 'suction method' – although it is unclear why, since no suction is involved. All other operations are performed via an abdominal incision.

  Because the womb is only about the size and shape of a small pear it can be freed from its surrounding tissue and supporting ligaments and taken out through the vagina. Although this operation requires considerable skill, it is the least traumatic for the woman. It is used to treat prolapse of the womb*, but cannot be carried out if the womb is enlarged due to large fibroids* or when it has adhered to other structures in the pelvis, as often happens in PID*.

SUB-TOTAL HYSTERECTOMY

Sub-total hysterectomy removes only the womb, leaving the cervix in place at the top of the vagina. This operation is rarely done now because if the cervix is left it would still be possible to develop cancer there. Some women, however, feel strongly about removal of the cervix, and you can request that it be left. Regular cervical smear tests* would still be necessary, and there may continue to be very light periods, if the woman is not past the menopause.

TOTAL HYSTERECTOMY

Total hysterectomy removes the womb and cervix. This operation is carried out most often. It is used to treat large fibroids* and, prior to endometrial ablation*/resection*, it was the standard surgical treatment for severe menstrual disorders. Persistent cervical pre-cancer (CIN)* is treated this way. It may be used to cure severe endometriosis*, although sometimes a more extensive operation is needed where one or both ovaries are also removed.

TOTAL HYSTERECTOMY WITH BI-LATERAL SALPINGO-OOPHORECTOMY

This operation removes the womb, cervix, both ovaries and both Fallopian tubes (bi-lateral means 'both-sided' and salpingo-oophorectomy means 'removal of Fallopian tubes and ovaries'). It is used to treat cancer of the womb* or ovaries*. Severe, widespread endometriosis* or PID* can also necessitate it. Removal of both ovaries from a woman who is not past the menopause can bring on menopausal symptoms due to the loss of the ovarian hormone oestrogen, and there is more about this later. But if one ovary, or even part of an ovary, can be left, this usually supplies enough hormones to prevent menopausal symptoms. After the menopause, the ovaries virtually cease producing hormones, so their removal causes no symptoms. If a woman is past the menopause when she needs a hysterectomy, for whatever reason, her ovaries are likely to be removed anyway; this protects her from any possibility of developing ovarian cancer* later on.

EXTENDED OR WERTHEIM'S HYSTERECTOMY

This is only used to treat invasive (spreading) cancer of the cervix* or womb* (uterine cancer). It is the most major and least common operation. The womb, cervix and upper vagina are removed, plus the surrounding fatty tissue and the lymph nodes* in the pelvis, to which uterine or cervical cancer* spreads. In a woman under 40 with cervical cancer, the ovaries and Fallopian tubes may be left, but they are always removed if cancer of the womb is being treated. The Wertheim operation may be followed by a course of radiotherapy* and/or chemotherapy* (anti-cancer drugs); these treatments are explained later (see Chapter 17). Even though the cervix has been removed, it will still be necessary to have regular smear tests* taken from the vagina after cancer surgery of this kind.

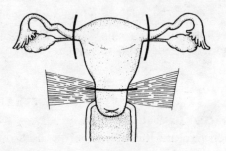

Types of abdominal hysterectomy
(1) Sub-total hysterectomy removes the womb, leaving the cervix and ovaries in place.

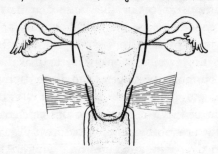

(2) Total hysterectomy removes the womb and cervix, leaving the ovaries. This operation may be done through either the vagina or abdomen.

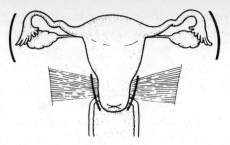

(3) Total hysterectomy with bi-lateral salpingo-oophorectomy removes the womb, cervix, both
    ovaries and both Fallopian tubes.

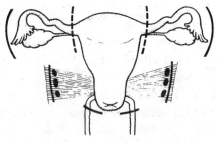

(4) Extended or Wertheim's hysterectomy is the most extensive operation, involving removal of
    the womb, cervix and upper vagina as well as surrounding tissue and lymph nodes. The
    ovaries and Fallopian tubes may be either removed or left.

What scars will I be left with after a hysterectomy?

If you have a vaginal hysterectomy, surgery is carried out
through the vagina and there will be no visible scars. After an
abdominal operation, you will have only a thin scar, which will
fade in time. The most usual incision is made just at the top of
the pubic hairline (a bikini incision). The hair needs to be
removed, of course, before the operation, but when it regrows
it will usually hide the scar.

Sometimes, however, it is necessary to make a vertical incision in the abdomen, from below the navel to the top of the
pubic hairline. Large fibroids* or an enlarged ovarian cyst* can
make this kind of incision necessary. This scar won't be hidden
by a bikini, but now that one-piece swimwear is just as fashion-
able and attractive, you don't need to worry. This incision is
used only when absolutely necessary.

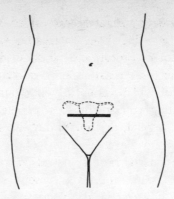

Position of incision for an abdominal hysterectomy. The scar will fade until it is scarcely noticeable.

When the womb is removed, what happens to the empty space left in the abdomen?

There is no empty space left in the abdomen after a hysterectomy. The intestines settle into the place which the womb occupied. This causes no problems.

Is there a hole at the top of the vagina if the womb and cervix have been removed?

No. The edges of the vagina are neatly stitched together at the top, using soluble stitches, which simply dissolve away during healing.

How are the ovaries and Fallopian tubes kept in place without the womb?

If the ovaries and Fallopian tubes are not removed during a hysterectomy, they are left in their natural positions, attached to their supporting tissues on the side walls of the pelvis, from which they also receive their blood supply.

Can you give me some advice on preparing for a hysterectomy?

Before going into hospital, read Chapter 2 of this book on Preparing for Surgery. Here is some advice specific to this operation.

One of the most important aspects of preparing for a hysterectomy is how you feel about it. Negative emotions are likely to make it more of an ordeal, and can slow down your recovery. As said earlier, emotional support is very important, as is understanding what will be done to you. Your own doctor and the specialist treating you are the best people to talk to about the operation. In hospital, the nurses can also help and reassure you. But they may not have the time to give you all the emotional support you need. Family, friends, and your partner, if you are in a relationship, can be a great source of strength.

Not everyone, however, can understand the physical and emotional impact an operation of this kind may have on you. It may be difficult, for instance, for a partner to come to terms with what is happening. Involving him, if possible, in the decision to have a hysterectomy can be very helpful to your relationship after surgery. Both of you are likely to be anxious about your recovery, your sex life, and whether there will be any long-term effects. If you visit your doctor or gynaecologist together and discuss your worries, this should help to allay your fears. Lend you partner this book, so he can read this chapter. Talk about the operation. The more you communicate, the better you will both cope.

Some men, however, just cannot relate to 'women's problems'. Or perhaps you are not in a relationship and are facing surgery on your own. Talking to a counsellor and to other women who have had hysterectomies can be very helpful in such situations. Your doctor or the hospital can put you in touch with a counsellor, and there may be a hysterectomy support group in your area which you can contact. Every woman's experience of hysterectomy is different, and it is worth hearing several accounts of what it is like, as well as discussing your own feelings. There are also books giving women's personal experiences of hysterectomy, some of which are listed in the References and Further Reading section of this book.

On a practical level, it is most important to be organized at home, because you will need time to recover from the operation. You will be in hospital for about 7 to 14 days, and it will take some weeks or months to recover, during which time you will be much less active than usual. Ensure that you will have enough help. If you will be returning to a family at home, impress upon them that you won't be fit in a mere two weeks; they must help out and not make demands on you. It will be very useful if you can stock up the freezer in advance. The less you have to worry about, the quicker you will recover.

What sort of state will I be in after the operation?

As with any major operation, you won't be feeling too good. This is how you are likely to be after a hysterectomy.

1. Immediately after the operation you will of course be drowsy. Your mouth will be dry. You may feel a bit sick from the anaesthetic, but will be given an injection if this is severe.

2. You will be on a drip*, which replaces fluid, as you won't be allowed to drink right away. If you need a blood transfusion*, this is given in the same way. Painkillers can also be given via a drip (or they can be injected into your buttock or thigh). This means that two or three slim tubes will be inserted into the veins in your hand or arm. These lead to bags containing the fluids, which are attached to a stand by the bed. In certain circumstances, painkillers may be given by epidural injection into the lower spine; see the question and answer on page 207.

3. There may be a drain from an abdominal incision; there is less likely to be one from the vagina after a vaginal hysterectomy. This slim tube carries away blood and other debris resulting from the operation. It leads to a bottle or bag under the bed, or to an absorbent pad on your abdomen, which is changed as necessary.

4. You may need a catheter – a tube in your urethra to help you urinate – which is also attached to a bottle or bag under the bed. This is more often inserted after a vaginal hysterectomy, but may not be necessary after an abdominal operation, unless you have difficulty urinating. It's

necessary to empty the bladder within 12 hours of the operation to prevent it from becoming over-distended; the nurses will ensure that you do pass water. A well-known way of encouraging it to happen naturally is to turn all the taps on in your ward or room.

5. If you're not expecting it, seeing these tubes can be a bit of a shock, but they are painless (although a drain or catheter may be a little uncomfortable). You may not need all of them anyway. They are removed within two to three days of the operation.

6. You will be wearing a sanitary towel and will have a light blood-stained discharge; this may go on for a few weeks after you have left hospital, and is normal. While it lasts, continue to wear sanitary towels, and not tampons, to reduce the risks of infection.

Will I be in a lot of pain?

A major operation is never a pleasant experience, although there is less discomfort following a vaginal hysterectomy than after an abdominal operation. But some of us are more sensitive to pain than others, and there's no need to suffer in silence – always say if you're in pain. Painkillers will be given after the operation by drip or injection as and when required. They can also be taken by mouth when your digestive system is working again, but since the digestive system 'shuts down' after an operation, especially an abdominal one, this may take a day or two.

As already mentioned, another method of giving pain relief is by epidural injection into the lower spine. A thin needle is inserted containing a fine polythene tube; painkillers are injected down it by syringe pump at the required rate. Insertion causes no discomfort because it is done while you are under anaesthetic. Given this way, painkillers don't make you at all drowsy. Unlike an epidural* in childbirth, this kind doesn't affect your bladder function or ability to move below the waist (it isn't used in childbirth because it is less effective for labour pains). It can be left in for two to three days. Its use is not standard practice after hysterectomy, but it is sometimes available.

Are there any 'alternative' or self-help methods of pain relief I could try?

Acupuncture can relieve pain and nausea. Although it is gaining ground as a worthwhile form of treatment, as yet very few hospitals offer it to patients. Meditation and relaxation techniques are self-help methods which can bring relief. Such 'alternative therapies' (see Chapter 18) can also be helpful when you are recovering at home. In any event, you should be over any severe pain before you leave hospital, and the nurses will do everything they can to make you comfortable, from giving pain relief to doing simple things, such as arranging your pillows to support you.

When will I get out of bed?

You will be helped out of bed and encouraged to walk around within a day or two; a nurse will carry the drip stand and you can be either detached from an epidural syringe or it can be carried, too. This may seem very soon to be out of bed, but it is essential to keep your circulation going and to prevent blood clots forming in your legs as a result of inactivity. If you have to stay in bed for any reason, you will need to do foot exercises or have your legs massaged. In certain circumstances anti-coagulant drugs may be given you to prevent blood clots.

After an abdominal operation you will find you can't stand up straight right away when you start walking, but don't worry about being 'bent over' – you'll straighten up as you heal. Your abdomen will be sore and you'll want to move carefully – it's very important not to put any strain on your abdominal muscles anyway, to avoid damaging the internal stitching.

Are there any ways I can make moving easier for myself?

Here are a couple of useful self-help techniques which will make moving easier at first and prevent you from putting any strain on your abdominal muscles.

1. To help yourself sit up and lie down in bed, you could take a strong cord into hospital which is long enough for

you to hold when it is tied to the foot of the bed (a man's dressing gown cord will do). You can pull yourself up and lower yourself on this.

2. Getting in and out of bed on your own won't be easy the first few times. The best way to do it is to roll onto your side with your knees bent up, then raise yourself on your elbow and swing your legs over the side of the bed, pushing yourself into a sitting position with your arms. To get back into bed, simply reverse the procedure; sit on the edge, lower yourself sideways using your arms and swing your legs up as you do this, then roll onto your back.

How soon will I be able to eat and drink?

You'll be allowed to drink the day following the operation and, usually, to eat the day after that. You probably won't be feeling hungry and solid food may not appeal – it's better to start with something soft and light, such as ice cream. Because the digestive system has been out of action, it won't function fully right away. Wind may build up, which can be very uncomfortable and cause your stomach to swell. This is common after hysterectomy, so don't be embarrassed about it. When you open your bowels, the wind will literally pass, although some women find it recurs. Drinking soda or peppermint water helps bring up wind, and the nurses can give you other remedies. Walking about also helps to get your digestive system working.

Are complications likely after hysterectomy?

About half the women who have hysterectomies will experience problems, but they can usually be resolved quite easily. Most common is infection; this isn't due to any medical negligence but because the vagina is not a sterile environment. Infection can be successfully treated with antibiotics; some gynaecologists give them routinely to guard against this.

A smelly, discoloured discharge, or heavy bleeding from the vagina, are signs of infection, although heavy bleeding soon after the operation can be due to a haemorrhage (a loss of blood) from the wound. If this happens, you may be in hospital for a few days longer and may need a blood transfusion*.

During a hysterectomy, the womb has to be cut away from the bladder, and this can make the area susceptible to infection. Pain or burning on urination are signs of this.

A haematoma (a blood clot) may form under an abdominal incision; this is rather like a bruise. It will be tender at first, but later will either be reabsorbed into the body during healing or be discharged through the wound: this may be rather alarming but in fact only requires gauze dressings until the discharge dries up spontaneously, usually after a few days.

Questions Women Most Often Ask About Hysterectomy

What advice can you give me on recovery?

Having a hysterectomy will be a different experience for each woman, and so will recovery. Some books provide step-by-step advice on the stages of recovery and how long each should take, usually up to a maximum of three months. Many women do recover fully in this time, and some even sooner, but others do not and may be made to feel pressurized or inadequate if they can't 'keep up' with a pre-ordained time-table.

The speed of recovery depends on such factors as your state of health before the operation and which operation you had: recovery after a vaginal hysterectomy is likely to be quicker than after a more extensive abdominal operation. If radiotherapy and/or chemotherapy treatment is given for cancer following surgery, this will also have an effect on recovery (see Chapter 17). Again, how much emotional support you receive and the amount of practical help you have afterwards play important roles in your in recovery. We can, however, give some helpful general guidelines.

1. Recovery usually begins while you are in hospital. After about the fifth day, you should start to feel better. The

stitches or clips are removed from an abdominal incision between the fifth and seventh day. Some surgeons use soluble stitches, which simply dissolve away. Before you leave hospital, you will be checked by your surgeon or a doctor to see that healing is progressing.

2. The hospital physiotherapist will explain the exercises you can do to help recovery. These will strengthen your internal pelvic floor muscles, which support your vagina, bladder and rectum; they are described on pages 112–13. Abdominal muscles tend to sag after surgery, and there are gentle exercises you can do to tone them, as illustrated. Start these as soon as you feel able, and do them every day, but stop if there is any pain.

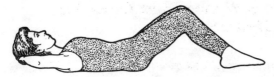

Gentle recovery exercises to firm and strengthen your abdominal muscles following surgery. To be carried out daily.

(1) Lie on your back, hands behind your head and elbows on the floor. Place feet and knees parallel about 30 cm (12 in) apart. Breathe in deeply.

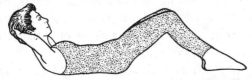

(2) Lift your head and shoulders off the floor a little, using your abdominal muscles, not your arms, until you can see your knees. Breathe out slowly as you lift and breathe in as you lower yourself back down. Repeat four times to start with.

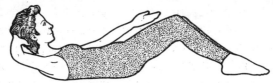

(3) Lifting your head and shoulders off the floor, reach through your knees with one hand, then repeat with the other hand. Breathe out as you reach forward, in as you release. Repeat four times. As you recover, increase the amount of exercise you do, but be guided by your physiotherapist's advice.

3   When you get home, tiredness may hit you hard for the first couple of weeks, and you are likely to feel fragile, nervous and low once you are away from the supportive hospital routine. Don't stay in bed, but rest at frequent intervals. Take short walks. Don't attempt any domestic chores. Alternatively, spend two weeks or so at a conva- lescent home (the hospital may be able to help with this) or at a quiet hotel, if there is someone who will go with you and it is within your budget.

4. Don't lift anything which strains your abdominal and pelvic floor muscles; internal healing takes time. This means no ironing, vacuuming, bedmaking or shopping for about five weeks, although you can do very light jobs (dusting, tidy- ing) before then. Don't stand for too long; invest in a high kitchen stool so you can sit to prepare vegetables or cook light meals when you feel able, but someone else must fetch and carry. Stop when you feel tired. Driving can strain internal muscles if you have to brake or swerve sud- denly, so only go out in the car as a passenger.

5. You will have been advised not to have sexual intercourse until you've had your post-op hospital check after six weeks, but this doesn't mean that lovemaking has to cease. There is advice on this and on restarting your sex life later in this chapter.

6. After your hospital check you should be able to resume most activities, including driving and light shopping (but no heavy lifting yet).

7. If you have a job, you should be able to go back to work between 8 and 12 weeks, if it is sedentary. After 12 weeks you may be able to resume your normal life. This means you can lift, but always do this correctly (see page 112). If you still tire easily, or feel psychologically 'knocked out', don't start feeling guilty.

8. Above all, listen to your body. It will tell you whether you are pushing yourself too much. You are likely to have good days and bad days throughout your convales- cence; try to do just that little bit more each week, but don't drive yourself to the point of exhaustion.

I've heard that women can get very depressed after a hysterectomy. How can I deal with this?

There is an ancient Greek myth which says that problems of the womb make women hysterical (morbidly or uncontrollably emotional, as defined in the dictionary), 'hustera' being Greek for womb. But any major operation is a shock to the system, and it's perfectly normal, whether you're a woman or a man, to react by feeling low for a short time afterwards, particularly when you first get home.

If you are well-prepared for a hysterectomy, you are less likely to become seriously depressed. If, however, you are very anxious about the operation, and feel anger or grief that this has happened to you, depression is more likely. Perhaps there are personal problems, such as relationship difficulties, which are being made worse by having a health problem. This is where counselling and emotional support can be so valuable.

Outside pressures can also cause depression – such as feeling that you haven't the time to be out of action for so long because of family or work commitments. But this is a time when you must put yourself first.

There can be entirely physical reasons for emotional upset. If your ovaries have been removed and you are not past the menopause, this can bring on a premature menopause due to a lack of the ovarian hormone oestrogen, as mentioned earlier. Depression and other menopausal symptoms can result.

If my ovaries are removed prior to the menopause, what symptoms will I experience?

It is important to find out beforehand whether your ovaries will indeed be removed. It's also important to discuss the possible effects, and what can be done about them, with your doctor or gynaecologist. Oestrogen is the hormone which supports fertility; the sudden loss after removal of the ovaries may cause stronger symptoms than a natural menopause, where hormone levels gradually drop as fertility ceases. Not all women have severe problems, however.

Menopausal symptoms can occur rapidly after surgery, or not for a few weeks or months. They are often a mixture of physical and psychological symptoms, and you should know what they are because otherwise they can be alarming.

Physical symptoms are:

- hot flushes/flashes; these come on suddenly and unexpectedly
- night sweats, which can be heavy and disturb sleep
- palpitations (racing heartbeat), which sometimes precede flushes or sweats
- frequent headaches
- itchy skin, as if insects are crawling under it
- vaginal dryness and soreness
- urinary problems

Psychological symptoms can include:

- irritability and mood swings
- loss of memory and ability to concentrate
- feelings of anxiety, which either have no obvious cause or are out of proportion to the cause
- loss of interest in sex
- constant fatigue

In the long term, oestrogen deficiency can lead to thinning of the bones (called osteoporosis) due to loss of calcium; this makes fractures more likely and causes the round-shouldered look sometimes seen in older women.

Can anything be done to relieve these symptoms?

Yes, the missing oestrogen can be replaced using hormone replacement therapy (HRT). This can be given in several forms: as a daily pill, as an implant under the skin of the thigh or abdomen, via a stick-on skin patch, or as a cream which is applied to the vagina. HRT is very effective in relieving menopausal symptoms and preventing the longer-term effects of oestrogen deficiency. Some women also consider that it improves the texture of their skin and hair, and generally counteracts the signs of ageing associated with the menopause.

Sometimes a hormone implant is inserted during a hysterectomy to guard against symptoms occurring afterwards. However, HRT may not be given until symptoms actually occur, and some doctors may want to wait even longer to see if the symptoms 'settle down' of their own accord. Even today, unfortunately, there are doctors who are reluctant to prescribe HRT at all. If you have severe symptoms and cannot get a sympathetic hearing from your doctor, see your gynaecologist or go to a 'well woman' clinic or to the menopause clinic of a hospital (see also the Useful Addresses section of this book).

If I am given HRT, how long do I need to take it for?

This varies, depending on your symptoms. The dose may also be adjusted to suit your needs. HRT may be needed for only a short time, but it can last several years, although breaks may be recommended to see whether your symptoms return. There is increasing evidence that long-term HRT may reduce the problem of osteoporosis in older women, as well as protecting against heart attacks and strokes. Much research is being carried out in this field of gynaecology.

Is HRT suitable for all women who have had their ovaries removed during a hysterectomy?

No, it is not suitable for all women. A thorough medical check is needed first. It cannot be prescribed for women who have had cancer of the womb, because it can promote the spread of the cancer. Although HRT does not cause uterine cancer, it is considered inadvisable to give any oestrogen if cancer has occurred. A woman who has had cervical or ovarian cancer* can have HRT. But if a woman has had breast cancer*, or has a family history of the disease, she may be advised not to have HRT. Conditions which used to make HRT inadvisable, such as high blood-pressure, diabetes, liver and gall bladder problems, need not be an obstacle if HRT is carefully given.

What should I do if I have menopausal symptoms after a hysterectomy but am unable to take HRT?

There are drugs which will relieve severe symptoms in the short term, but you may want to try remedies such as taking vitamins C, D and E – and evening primrose oil, which some women find helps with flushes and sweats. Regular exercise will promote bone strength, and a balanced diet can do much to increase energy. Read Chapter 18 on Alternative Therapies and Healthier Living.

Will I continue to have a 'menstrual cycle' after a hysterectomy where my ovaries have not been removed?

Yes, if you are not past the menopause. You will still have the 'feelings' you had during your menstrual cycle before your hysterectomy, such as mid-cycle ovulation* pain and breast tenderness before a period, although you won't have periods without a womb, of course. You will go through a natural menopause, but without the menstrual symptoms of irregular periods or periods ceasing. You may need HRT then.

Why do women put on weight after a hysterectomy?

It's easy for women to gain weight during convalescence after a hysterectomy because it's necessary to be so much less active. A healthy diet which avoids sugary and starchy foods will prevent weight gain, speed recovery and help your self-image after surgery. Keeping yourself mentally occupied will distract you from thoughts of food. Convalescence is an opportunity to do such things as catching up on reading, listening to music and watching videos of those films you missed. Conversation is also a good mental stimulus. But a woman who becomes very much overweight may be suffering from depression and is eating as a way of trying to cheer herself up, although putting on weight usually has the opposite effect. This is when counselling may be needed. There is no reason why the operation itself should cause weight gain.

Exercise is important, too, in preventing weight gain and in helping you to become fully active. You can start with short walks right away. Following your post-op check, you will probably be able to take more exercise. Swimming is particularly good, because the whole body is exercised while being supported by water, so there is no stress or jarring. But don't jump or dive in right away; find out what your body can take first. Cycling is also good gentle exercise after hysterectomy.

I'm worried about the effect hysterectomy will have on my sex life.

Much depends on what your relationship with your partner was like before surgery. If it was close and loving, the chances are that it will continue to be so after hysterectomy. And if the operation has cured a problem which interfered with sex by causing discomfort or pain, your sex life is likely to be much improved.

A partner's loving support can be very important, particularly during convalescence. You will have been advised not to have intercourse before your post-op hospital check, but during this time sexual pleasuring without penetration can be physically and emotionally very reassuring. Caressing, oral sex and mutual masturbation are all possible. Couples for whom lovemaking is about penetration may need to learn to enjoy these other forms of pleasuring; there are some helpful sex manuals listed in the References and Further Reading section.

When you restart intercourse, your partner will need to be gentle and to pace lovemaking slowly, because your arousal may take longer. If your ovaries have been removed before the menopause, vaginal dryness and soreness can make intercourse difficult. HRT or a lubricating jelly will help. Radiotherapy* can cause the vagina to stiffen and shrink, but gentle intercourse with a lubricant stretches it, thus counteracting these problems. If the vagina has been shortened by surgery, gentle intercourse with partial penetration is still possible.

Some women experience a loss of libido (desire) after hysterectomy. This may be because the pelvic area has become less sensitive. Sensitivity should return; this can be helped by doing pelvic floor exercises (see page 112). Alternatively, it may be due to the removal of the ovaries; these also secrete androgens – hormones which stimulate sexual arousal. Androgens can be replaced, like oestrogen, but at the present time can only be given via an implant. Other methods of replacing these hormones are being researched. However, sexual arousal depends as much on the mind as the body. If either partner has fears about sex following hysterectomy, or if there are relationship problems, lack of desire is often the result. Below are questions on some common worries.

Is there any danger that intercourse will damage the scar at the top of my vagina?

No, it won't damage the scar. If there is a little bleeding after sex this is probably because granules of tissue have developed around the scar, which is quite common, and they can be removed easily and painlessly by a doctor. Some women enjoy having the scar stretched during intercourse and find that their vagina seems to have been pleasurably tightened by the operation. Others say they feel slacker inside, which is likely to be because the pelvic muscles need toning, rather than because the vagina really is looser.

Will I still be able to have orgasms?

Yes. The 'trigger' for orgasm is the clitoris – the small protrusion above the urethral opening. This is unaffected by surgery. Stimulating the clitoris by hand or through close body contact during intercourse will still bring about orgasm. It may feel different because the womb is no longer involved in the repeated muscular contractions of orgasm. Some women say the sensation is sharper.

time, you should ultimately feel that a hysterectomy was necessary and worthwhile.

Is there any medical progress towards making a hysterectomy a less traumatic operation?

New methods using a laparoscope* are being developed for carrying out pelvic operations, including hysterectomy. Using laparoscopy* would turn a major operation, such as a hysterectomy, into a relatively minor procedure for the patient because an abdominal incision would no longer be needed. Great surgical skill would be required, however, because the surgeon would be operating via small incisions in the abdomen and using very fine instruments to remove the organs. Although it may be some time before such procedures are in general use, they do hold out much hope for the future.

16

BREAST SURGERY

A woman's breasts are vital to her self-image, being uniquely feminine. The possibility of breast disease which requires surgery causes all women great fear and distress. Finding a lump in the breast is a dreaded event which provokes thoughts of pain, mutilation and death. Yet the vast majority of these lumps turn out to be benign and may only require treatment by simple procedures which leave the breast intact.

Disfiguring surgery is by no means always needed now for breast cancer, which can be very successfully treated, especially if caught early. In this chapter the treatment options for breast cancer are explained. We also explain how you can help yourself by increasing your overall 'breast awareness' and by having medical checks, so that if there are any problems, they can be diagnosed and treated without delay.

How will increasing my overall 'breast awareness' help me to detect any problems?

Greater importance is being placed on women familiarizing themselves with their breasts, starting in their teens when breast problems of any kind are rare. The texture of normal breasts can vary at different times of the month. For instance, breasts are more likely to be tender and to feel uneven in the second half of the menstrual cycle before a period. Knowing what is 'normal' for you will help you to detect any changes which are unusual so that you can report them to your doctor promptly.

I'm not sure what is 'normal' for me, and the idea of 'looking for trouble' worries me.

Have a check-up with your doctor, who can reassure you about the health of your breasts. You can then start familiarizing yourself with them, knowing that they are normal. This should help you overcome any unnecessary anxieties you may have about what is or is not normal for you. It's a matter of monitoring your breast health in a positive way, rather than of 'looking for trouble'.

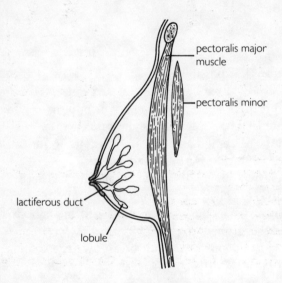

pectoralis major
muscle

pectoralis minor

lactiferous duct

lobule

A normal breast: the lobules (milk-producing glands), the lactiferous (milk) ducts, and the chest muscles.

Take whatever opportunities occur in your daily life to check your breasts, such as during a bath or shower, while applying body lotion, or when dressing. This is particularly important for women over 40. Know the kind of changes to look for: these are given in the captions to the illustrations on page 223 and earlier in the book (see page 8).

Recommendations on breast self-examination – how and when to carry it out – can vary, depending on the country in which you live. Follow the advice given by your doctor on self-

examination. If you are recommended to use the technique
illustrated, ensure that your doctor or a health care professional
teaches you how to carry it out correctly; the illustrations here
are a guide to the technique. Self-examination and overall
'breast awareness' cannot replace medical checks, which you
should have as often as your doctor advises.

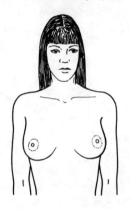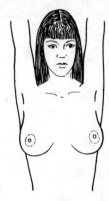

A guide to self-examination.
(1) *Stand with your arms by your sides and, in a good light, look at your breasts in a mirror.
    Look for any changes, such as:*
    - *differences in the size of either breast*
    - *inverted or cracked nipples, or the nipple 'pulling' to one side*
    - *dimpled or discoloured skin on the breast*
    - *a rash on the breast or nipple*
(2) *Raise your arms above your head and look again. This will emphasize any differences in the
    breasts.*

If early diagnosis of breast cancer is so important, are there any ways of
detecting it before a lump can be felt?

Yes. Mammography is a form of X-ray* which can detect
tumours no bigger than a pinpoint. The earlier cancer is diagnosed, the less likely it is to have spread to other parts of the
body. In Britain, it's recommended as a routine screening procedure for all women over 50 and for some women over 40 who
may be more at risk of developing breast cancer (see page 231
for information). However, the precise age at which routine
screening of all women starts varies in different countries.

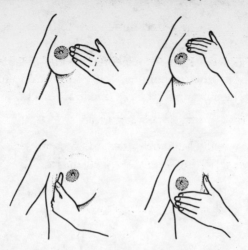

(3) Lie flat on your back with your head supported comfortably on a pillow (placing a folded towel under the side you are going to examine first spreads the breast tissue and makes examination easier). Feel the right breast with your left hand using the flat of your fingers. Starting at the nipple, work your fingers over the whole breast, using small, circular movements and firm but gentle pressure. Repeat for the left breast, using your right hand.

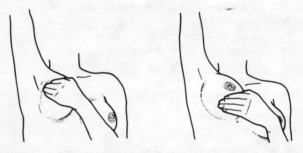

(4) Raise your arm above your head and examine each whole breast again, right up into your armpit. Note any unusual thickening or lumps, and if you find any, report them to your doctor without delay.

Mammography is not helpful for younger women because the breast tissue is too dense; breast cancer is also much less usual in younger age groups. Ultrasound* may be used to detect cancer in younger women, but is not a routine screening method. It can also show whether breast lumps are solid or contain fluid (cysts).

If I find a lump what should I do?

Stay calm, don't jump to any conclusions, and see your doctor right away.

Won't benign lumps go away of their own accord?

Some of them will, but you must not wait to see if this will happen before reporting a lump to your doctor.

How do benign lumps differ from cancer? Do they ever turn malignant?

Benign tumours behave quite differently to cancer. They may increase in size but, unlike cancer, they don't invade surrounding healthy tissue or spread to other parts of the body. Very rarely do they ever turn malignant.

Is there any way I can tell if a lump is malignant?

No, not for sure. A cancerous lump can sometimes mimic a benign one, and vice versa; there is more on this later.

What will happen if I report a breast lump to my doctor?

Read Chapter 1 on Diagnosing Women's Problems, which describes how the doctor will carry out a breast examination. Doctors will treat a lump as cancerous until proven otherwise, and you will be referred to a specialist very quickly. In the UK, breast problems are usually treated by a general surgeon with a specialization in breast disease; in other countries they are the province of a gynaecologist. When you are referred to a general surgeon, this doesn't mean you are bound to have an operation. But further tests may be needed to find out the nature of the lump. As most lumps are benign, we'll start with their treatment.

Could you describe the different kinds of benign lumps and what can be done about them?

BENIGN MAMMARY DYSPLASIA

BMD is the most common cause of breast lumps or lumpiness in women aged 30 to 50. It usually affects both breasts, and also causes tenderness. Symptoms are more severe in the second half of the menstrual cycle, but in some women they may go away following a period, which is why BMD is also called cyclical mastalgia. It has several other names, so if you hear it called something different, it still refers to the same thing; these are fibroadenosis, chronic or cystic mastitis, fibrocyctic disease and benign breast disease.

BMD most often affects the upper, outer parts of the breast. There may be diffused, small cysts, or just one or two large ones. Women with irregular periods, or who have no children, are more prone to BMD. It is thought to be related to fluctuating hormones, particularly a high level of oestrogen (a hormone produced by the ovaries). Although there is no definite association with cancer, regular medical checks are especially important, as it is necessary to establish that BMD is not masking early breast cancer. A woman with BMD should also get to know her 'usual' lumps and bumps, so she can report any changes to her doctor promptly. But she is no more likely to get cancer because she has BMD.

Removal

Removal or other treatment is not generally needed; BMD may resolve itself in time, and will disappear after the menopause. A low-fat diet may help because body fat is thought to raise oestrogen levels (see page 269). Taking evening primrose oil may also help balance hormones. The combined oral contraceptive pill can both prevent and relieve BMD because it 'evens out' hormone levels. If BMD is very severe, more powerful drugs can be prescribed, but these have side-effects, and only relatively few women will need them. Larger cysts can be aspirated (emptied); see below.

CYSTS

Cysts are very common benign breast lumps. They may occur singly or be part of BMD. These fluid-filled sacs may be found in any part of the breast; their cause is unknown. They can vary in size from very small to about 5 cm (2 in) across. Usually painless, they feel smooth and can be moved around with the fingers. There is no connection between cysts and breast cancer.

Removal

This is done by needle aspiration, which can be performed without anaesthetic – all you will feel is a small prick, as when a blood sample is taken. After a cyst has been drained, the lump will have gone. This is an out-patient procedure, there are no after-effects and you can go home straight away. However, if you've had a cyst, another may occur, in which case it would also be aspirated if it didn't disperse of its own accord.

FIBROADENOMA

A fibroadenoma is a hard, smooth, well-defined lump, just like a marble, which is painless and can be anything from 1 to 3 cm (½ to 1½ in) in size. It is also called a 'breast mouse' because it slips around under your fingers when you feel it. Common in young women up to about the age of 25, its cause is unknown. In the past, it was always removed, but nowadays many surgeons are prepared to leave small fibroadenomas in women aged less than 25 years, provided the patient is happy with this decision.

Removal

Removing a fibroadenoma involves a minor operation which can be done under local or general anaesthetic. An incision of about 2 cm (1 in) is made, usually near the areola which surrounds the nipple, and the lump excised. The incision is then stitched. If it's carried out under a local anaesthetic in the out-patient department of a hospital, you can go home right away. For a general anaesthetic, you may be in hospital overnight. You probably won't need painkillers afterwards. Wear a soft supporting bra for comfort during healing. The stitches can be removed by your doctor or at the hospital within a week. The scar will fade until it is scarcely noticeable. There are absolutely no after-effects; the breast looks the same and you will be able to breastfeed.

DUCT PAPILLOMAS

The first symptom of these is a yellowish or blood-stained discharge from the nipple. They are little warty protrusions that grow in the lactiferous (milk-producing) ducts under the nipple. Gently pressing the nipple area during self-examination may enable you to feel papillomas; pressure may also produce the discharge. They can occur at any age, but are much less common after the menopause; why they occur is unknown. There is a slight tendency for them to turn malignant, so removal is necessary.

Removal

This is minor surgery under general anaesthetic. A small incision is made at the side of the nipple and the duct(s) containing the papillomas removed; this will not affect your ability to breast-feed. As for fibroadenoma removal, you would be in hospital for only a day or two, discomfort would be minimal, and stitches removed within a week. The breast is left intact, with only a very small scar. Again, wearing a soft supporting bra during healing will be more comfortable.

DUCT ECSTASIA

This a common cause of breast pain which tends to affect women over 40. The lactiferous ducts fill with fluid and become blocked and inflamed. A soft, uneven lump or lumps form and can be felt under the areola. There is a nipple discharge (watery, blood-stained, brown or greenish), and after a while the nipple may retract. As with some other benign problems, why this occurs in unknown. It often settles down without treatment, beyond the woman taking aspirin or paracetamol to relieve discomfort. Sometimes antibiotics can help. Duct ecstasia has no connection with malignancy, but if there is a continuing problem, surgery which removes the ducts may be needed in a few cases.

Removal

Removal of ducts is done in hospital under general anaesthetic, requiring a stay of one or two days. An incision is made round the areola and a cone-shaped segment of tissue containing the ducts is removed from under the nipple. The nipple is then stitched back in place. It causes discomfort and soreness, so painkillers will be needed. The breast will be a bit less rounded and the nipple flatter afterwards. Breastfeeding wouldn't be possible from this breast, but a woman with the problem is likely to be past her childbearing years anyway. Stitches are removed in a week. If your bra presses on the nipple you may be more comfortable without one while you are healing. Duct ecstasia cannot recur after treatment.

ABSCESS

An abscess can form in the breast during breastfeeding. Although it's not particularly common, it is more likely to occur in the month after a first baby is born. Infection can enter via a cracked nipple, and this leads to inflammation. It has no connection with breast cancer. If infection is diagnosed at an early stage, when there is simply a red, sore area, taking antibiotics can cure it. But if the area is allowed to become hot, tense, swollen and throbbingly painful (the woman may also have a fever and chills), pus will have formed, which needs releasing; antibiotics on their own won't be sufficient.

Removal

Removal may sometimes be possible by needle aspiration: the pus is sucked out using a hollow needle inserted in the breast. This is done under local anaesthetic at a hospital out-patient clinic. Antibiotics will then clear the infection.

Usually, minor surgery will be necessary. This is carried out under general anaesthetic in hospital, and you would probably be in overnight. An incision is made and the abscess opened and drained. A small drainage tube is left in place for a few days afterwards, so the incision is not stitched. The tube drains into a gauze dressing on the breast and you can go home with it in place. None of this is painful – the operation will have brought rapid relief from pain – but the woman may worry that she will be left with a hole or large scar. This is not the case. Healing is rapid and, although there will be a small scar, there is no indentation left, nor are there any long-term effects.

Abscesses can be prevented by not allowing the breasts to become engorged (over-filled); feed the baby more often, or express surplus milk by hand or with a breast pump. Clean and dry the nipples after feeding, and apply a soothing cream such as lanolin. Using a nipple guard during breastfeeding may prevent cracking.

FAT NECROSIS

This is a lump which forms as the result of an injury – a severe bump or blow to the breast. You would certainly remember how it happened because you would have experienced immediate pain and bruising. Necrosis means 'death of cells', caused by fat cells bursting open upon impact. The body reacts by forming scar tissue round the injured area; this creates a hard, irregular lump. The scar tissue tends to contract, pulling on the ligaments in the breast and causing a dimpling of the skin over the lump. Although it resembles cancer, a fat necrosis is never cancerous, but it may explain why women with breast cancer often believe it started with an injury. Most likely, it was the injury which led them to check their breasts for the first time and find the cancerous lump that was already there. Breast cancer does not result from an injury, and fat necrosis is a rare type of lump.

Removal

Removal is the same as for fibroadenoma. It is usually carried out because fat necrosis may mimic malignancy.

If there is little or no connection between benign lumps and breast cancer, what causes it?

The precise cause or causes of breast cancer are unknown. But like all cancers, it develops when something happens to damage cells and make their normal functioning go haywire. Instead of dividing to replace old cells which die, they multiply out of control to produce a growth (lump or tumour) which, as already mentioned, invades surrounding healthy tissue.

Malignant cells break off from the growth and travel to other parts of the body, where they form 'secondary' growths, or metastases. It is these, rather than the primary tumour, which are more difficult to treat. Hence, again, the importance of early diagnosis of primary tumours in the breast.

You said that some women may be more at risk of developing breast cancer. What does this mean, and am I likely to be one of them?

Breast cancer is, unfortunately, on the increase, but this may be because women generally are living longer and it tends to affect older age groups. A recent report in the USA states that as many as 1 in 10 women are likely to get the disease. Although the precise causes are unknown, it is associated with certain factors. The main ones are listed here.

- A woman is more likely to develop breast cancer in her 50s than at any other age. This doesn't mean you're nec-essarily more at risk just through being this age – it sim-ply means you need to be particularly vigilant at this time of life.
- Women whose periods began early (under 12) or who had a late menopause (over 50) seem to be slightly more at risk.
- Not having any children, or having them over the age of 25, slightly increases the risk. Early childbearing and breastfeeding do appear to have some protective effect.
- The strongest single risk factor is a family history of breast cancer (but not other types of cancer), i.e. if a sis-ter, mother, aunt or grandmother has had breast cancer. The risk is mostly increased in women who have a mother or sister who developed cancer before the age of 50. This isn't to say it's definitely hereditary, but it does seem to run in families. These are the women who would be rec-ommended to have early screening.
- Women generally in Western Europe, the USA and Australasia are at greater risk than women in Eastern Europe, the Far East and the developing world,

irrespective of family history. The high-fat Western diet is increasingly suspect. This is because when women from a country such as Japan (where there is a low-fat diet and a low risk of breast cancer) live in the West and adopt the diet, their risk becomes the same.

- Being very overweight is an associated factor, especially in older women.

Are these risk factors linked in any way?

It is thought they could be. The female hormone oestrogen, produced by the ovaries, is known to play a part in stimulating the growth of certain tumours. Early menstruation, childlessness – or delayed childbearing – and late menopause all have one thing in common: they allow prolonged exposure to high levels of oestrogen, which would be interrupted by early childbearing and breastfeeding. Because women in the Western world are well-nourished, they start menstruating early and have a late menopause; they also tend to put off having children into their late 20s and early 30s, and sometimes beyond that.

Women who eat lots of fatty foods (the Western diet) are found to have higher oestrogen levels because body fat produces oestrogen independently of the ovaries. Very overweight women therefore have higher oestrogen levels than slim ones; this is probably a factor in their having a greater risk of breast cancer after the menopause, when oestrogen levels would normally drop.

But women who are apparently without such risk factors can still develop breast cancer.

Isn't radiation a risk factor? I'm worried that the X-rays used in mammography could actually promote breast cancer.

Excessive exposure to radiation does increase the chances of breast and other cancers. But nowadays the dose of X-rays given for a mammogram is minimal and there is virtually no risk. However, when carefully measured and targeted, X-rays can also be a powerful weapon in treating cancer by radiotherapy*.

I've been advised to have mammography, but somehow I don't really want it.

Some women are reluctant to face the possibility that 'something serious' might be found. If they feel well, mammography may seem unnecessary anyway, but you don't have to feel ill to have breast cancer. Among their fears may be anxiety about the disruption cancer will bring to their lives and the lives of those close to them. They'd just rather not know. It can only be repeated that if anything is wrong, then the sooner it is 'caught' the less trauma there will be.

I'm having a mammogram. How is it carried out, and will it hurt?

It will be done in a 'well woman' or hospital out-patient clinic. If you have had previous X-rays, take them along for comparison. You need to undress to the waist and stand or sit close to the machine. Each breast will be X-rayed in turn. This is done by gently compressing the breast between an X-ray plate below, which picks up the image, and a plastic cover above. This can be uncomfortable but it is not painful. In a routine mammogram, one image of each breast is usually taken. The radiographer will go behind a screen, just as happens in a dental X-ray, because s/he carries out so many mammograms that protection is needed, although the risk to you is negligible. You will receive the results from your doctor in about a week. Occasionally, you may be recalled for further views to be taken, but this doesn't necessarily mean you have cancer. Mammograms are not always easy to interpret. Another method of carrying out mammography is to X-ray the breast from the side as it hangs freely. This may be particularly necessary for small-breasted women.

How can they tell whether or not I have cancer?

Cancerous growths often contain deposits of calcium, and these show up white on a mammogram, although a biopsy* (removal of a sample of tissue, or the whole tumour) is always needed to verify this. A biopsy is carried out whether a tumour is discovered by mammogram or self-examination.

What will happen next if cancer is diagnosed? I find it hard to imagine such an appalling event.

It is of course a terrible shock to be told you have breast cancer, particularly if you don't actually feel ill, as is often the case. Some hospitals may provide a specially trained nurse counsellor who will be present when you are told and who will be available to advise and help you in every possible way during and after treatment. You may want to have someone with you who is close to you when you are told. But some doctors feel it is better if they are able to break the news, and help you come to terms with it, on a one-to-one basis. Or they may have other specialists at hand who will be involved in your treatment, and who can also advise and reassure you.

How is breast cancer treated?

This depends on the stage it has reached.

Could you give some more information about the disease?

There are different types of breast cancer. The most common kind occurs in the cells of milk ducts. Less commonly, it may be found in the lobules (the milk-producing glands). Cancer in other sites is even rarer. If it is described as a carcinoma in situ, this means it hasn't yet invaded surrounding healthy tissue. The outlook is very good if it is caught and treated at this earliest stage. Breast X-rays may detect carcinoma in situ before any lump is present.

When a cancer becomes invasive, the first symptom which can be detected by hand is an irregular, painless lump, but occasionally the cancer may be smooth. Most often, it appears in the upper, outer quarter of the breast, although it can occur elsewhere. (It is very unusual for both breasts to be affected at once.) At this stage, the lump can be moved with the fingers.

Further invasion causes the tumour to pull on the ligaments in the breast, which produces a dimple in the skin. Any spread along the ducts shrinks them and this inverts the nipple or pulls it to one side.

As cancer spreads, the tumour becomes fixed to the skin above and the chest muscles below. It may produce excessive fluid, which causes the skin over the lump to thicken and develop an orange-peel texture.

The axillary lymph nodes* in the armpit will harden and swell if cancer cells have invaded them. The lymph nodes are vital to the body's immune system (our natural defence against disease); if they have lost the battle against the disease, it can spread to other parts of the body via the lymphatic system and the bloodstream. It can develop anywhere, but tends to favour the lungs, liver and bones. Blood tests, further X-rays or a CT scan* (a 'whole body' X-ray) can show whether there are 'secondaries' elsewhere.

From the descriptions we have given of benign and malignant tumours, you can see why you shouldn't jump to any conclusions – and why early diagnosis is so essential.

What are the treatments for breast cancer?

Before any treatment is carried out, your specialist should discuss the options thoroughly with you. There is no rigid course of treatment; specialists can differ in their approaches and you must feel convinced you understand and agree with the treatment recommended. Some women prefer it if the specialist decides what is best for them; others want to be part of the decision-making process. If necessary, take a couple of weeks to think about the proposed treatment – the cancer won't advance significantly in that time. Talk to the nurse counsellor, if the hospital provides one. Some of the well-known cancer charities have advisory services and can put you in touch with other women who have had treatment. You may find that well-meaning friends and relatives offer confusing advice. While you need all the emotional support you can get, rely on the medical experts for medical advice. But if you have any doubts about treatment which can't be resolved with your specialist, you can ask your doctor to refer you to another specialist.

How are the treatments carried out?

The general approach to the treatment of breast cancer is to carry out as little surgery as possible, depending on the size of the cancer. This has been found to be no less effective than the more extensive and mutilating operations of the past.

LUMPECTOMY

Lumpectomy is usual for many early breast cancers. This simply involves removing the lump, together with a margin of healthy tissue. It causes little, if any, distortion to the shape of the breast and leaves only a small, thin scar. Some lymph nodes* may be removed from the armpit via a separate incision to check whether or not cancer cells have spread to them.

QUADRANTECTOMY

This is a variation of lumpectomy, where the lump and a larger segment of surrounding tissue are removed. The effects of this surgery show more in small-breasted women.

SUBCUTANEOUS MASTECTOMY

This involves removal of all the breast tissue, leaving the skin and nipple intact. An incision is made under the breast and tissue removed through it. The breast can then be reconstructed using an implant. See page 243 for more information on breast reconstruction.

SIMPLE MASTECTOMY

A simple mastectomy removes all the breast tissue, and may be carried out when cancer cells are more widespread but still confined to the breast. After the operation the chest is flat and the incision heals leaving a thin scar across it. This is not necessarily a permanent state: breast reconstruction may be possible.

RADICAL MASTECTOMY

This is the most extensive operation performed today. The breast and the lymph nodes* in the armpit are completely removed, together with the smaller chest muscle, called the pectoralis minor, which underlies the main pectoralis major muscle. This is done to clear all the lymph nodes in the chest. There is a thin scar across the chest and into the armpit. Breast reconstruction may be possible after this operation, too.

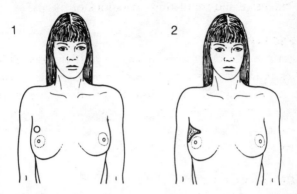

Surgery for breast cancer.
(1) Lumpectomy: removal of lump only, plus a margin of healthy tissue. This leaves only a small scar.
(2) Quadrantectomy: the lump and a larger segment of tissue are removed. This will be more obvious in smaller-breasted women.

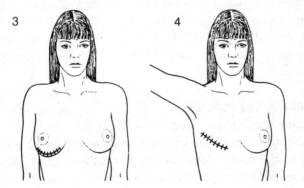

(3) Subcutaneous mastectomy: removal of all the breast tissue via an incision under the breast, leaving the skin and nipple intact to allow for reconstruction using an implant.
(4) Simple mastectomy: removal of the entire breast, leaving a thin scar across the chest. Reconstruction may still be possible.

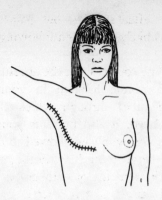

(5) *Radical mastectomy: the most extensive operation; this leaves a thin scar which extends into the armpit. Reconstruction may still be possible.*

What preparations would I need to make before surgery?

See Chapter 2 on Preparing for Surgery for the basic general information. If you are having a lumpectomy you will be in hospital for only about three days and recovery will be swift. However, you will probably need a course of radiotherapy* to ensure that any remaining cancer cells in the breast are 'killed off'. This treatment requires regular visits to a hospital radiotherapy clinic, and can be very tiring. So, before you go into hospital, ensure that you have transport and enough help at home for the weeks to come.

For a more extensive operation, you will be in hospital for at least a week and recovery will take some weeks or months. It may be followed by radiotherapy* and/or chemotherapy* (anti-cancer drugs). Again, arrange to have enough help at home. This is where a cancer charity or support group can often be particularly helpful both in giving emotional reassurance and providing practical assistance.

What will it be like after surgery? Will I be in a lot of pain?

Lumpectomy is not a painful operation, nor is mastectomy reckoned to be among the more painful operations, but we all have a different level of sensitivity to pain. Some women experience a burning sensation after surgery, but painkillers are always given. This is what is likely to happen following a mastectomy.

1. When you 'come round' from the anaesthetic you may be on a drip (a needle inserted in your hand or arm, attached to a tube) through which fluid lost during surgery is replaced; it also prevents you from becoming dehydrated, as you won't be allowed to drink right away. Painkillers can be given in this way too, or by injection.

2. If you feel sick from the anaesthetic an injection can be given to quell nausea, if it is severe. You won't be given anything to eat straight away, but you probably won't feel like it anyway. Your digestive system needs time to get back into action following the anaesthetic.

3. There will be a drain* from the incision (and from under the arm if the lymph nodes* have been removed) to clear any liquid debris following surgery (you may also have a slim tube in place following a lumpectomy). These tubes drain into bottles. The tubes will be removed within a few days and are just pulled out, which shouldn't hurt.

4. There's no need to stay in bed, and you will be encouraged to sit out and walk around as soon as possible. A nurse will carry the drip stand if necessary; the drainage bottles will also have to travel with you, prior to removal of the tubes. An easy way of arranging this is to put them in plastic shopping bags and carry these.

5. The incision will be covered by a dressing and needs to be kept dry for about a week. You can have a bath, provided you don't get the dressing wet.

6. The hospital physiotherapist will visit you and give you exercises to do; these will help you regain strength in your arm and shoulder. You won't damage the stitches or incision by doing them. Before you leave the hospital, your arm should be strong enough to enable you to comb your hair and fasten clothes at the back.

7. Stitches or clips are removed within 10 days; this is carefully done and is not painful. If a reconstruction was carried out, seeing your 'new' breast may come as a relief.

More often, however, reconstruction is carried out later. Seeing a mastectomy incision for the first time will inevitably be a shock. A nurse counsellor may be present, as well as your surgeon. Although the incision will still be red (it fades with healing) it will be neat. Women often have difficulty looking at themselves after a mastectomy, and time may be needed for them to do this. Seeing the incision in a mirror for the first time may make it easier, because this is somehow less immediate.

8. The hospital will provide a soft, lightweight, temporary prosthesis (false breast) for you to wear inside your bra until healing is complete. There's a variety of permanent prostheses available to suit all shapes and sizes, so your figure will look as it did before when you are dressed. The incision will be placed so it won't show if you wear low-cut clothes; you can sew a prosthesis into a sports bra or swimwear, so there's no risk of it coming adrift during vigorous exercise. But not all women want to wear one – some find it easier to accept what has happened by not disguising the result. It is entirely the woman's choice.

Can you give me some idea of the physical and emotional after-effects?

Many women quite rightly feel elated straight after surgery; they've 'come through' and coped well – often better than they thought they would. In hospital, the staff and very often other patients can be most supportive and encouraging. But after returning home, it's easy to become depressed. Part of this is simply normal fatigue following surgery. But grief at the loss of a breast and fears about cancer recurring usually surface now. This is of course when the support of loved ones, your doctor and surgeon, and perhaps a cancer charity or support group, can be most valuable.

Physically, healing should progress without complications. The area may feel numb, although some women have 'phantom' feelings, as if their breast was still there. It's usual for the skin to thicken during healing, so don't worry about this. Healing may be helped by applying a soothing calendula cream, made from marigolds. If there is any sign of redness or soreness it should be reported to your doctor, as there may be an infection, which can be treated successfully with antibiotics.

Could you say more about the post-op exercises I may need to do?

If your lymph nodes* have been removed, your arm and shoulder may swell. This is due to accumulated fluid (lymph) which is normally dispersed by the nodes but now needs to find new channels. Arm and shoulder exercises can help this and will enable you to regain strength if your pectoralis minor muscle has been removed. A particularly helpful one is where you 'walk' your hands up a wall. This simply involves standing facing a wall and then 'walking' your hands up it as far as you can without causing pain. Aim to get a bit higher each day. It should be possible to restore arm movement completely, so that you can even play a sport such as tennis.

Should swelling persist, sleep with your arm raised on a pillow. During the day, sit with it resting on the back of your chair. You may need to wear an elastic sleeve. Resistance to infection can be reduced in the arm, so be careful not to cut yourself when shaving under your arms or during a manicure. Always wear gloves when doing housework or gardening.

Can you give me some advice on radiotherapy and chemotherapy?

Before you leave hospital your surgeon will explain the results of tests on the tumour that was removed, and will discuss any treatment with radiotherapy and/or chemotherapy which may be necessary.

In some hospitals, a radioactive implant may be placed in the breast when a lumpectomy is performed, or sometimes after a course of external radiotherapy has been carried out.

External radiotherapy can be started when healing is complete, and may be used on the primary tumour site and elsewhere on the body if cancer has spread.

Like external radiotherapy, chemotherapy is an out-patient treatment which may be spread over several weeks or months.

Powerful anti-cancer drugs are given by mouth or injection. Chemotherapy for breast cancer today does not usually cause severe side-effects. Tamoxifen is the drug most often used because it blocks oestrogen and inhibits the spread of cancer. It's taken in tablet form and may bring on menopausal symptoms* in a pre-menopausal woman, but does not prevent pregnancy (so contraception is still necessary, as you should not become pregnant during treatment for cancer). After the menopause, when the majority of women with breast cancer will be taking it, there are few side-effects. It can even be used to control breast cancer in elderly women if surgery is inadvisable.

Before tamoxifen became available, the ovaries were either removed or irradiated (bombarded with X-rays) to stop them producing oestrogen. Sometimes the adrenal glands above the kidneys were also removed, because they produce hormones thought to promote breast cancer, but now drugs have made this unnecessary.

The cytotoxic drugs, which act by killing cancer cells, are more likely to have side-effects, but these can often be controlled. See Chapter 17 for further information on radiotherapy and chemotherapy.

Is there any medical progress towards preventing breast cancer, apart from screening?

Yes. At the time of writing the drug tamoxifen is being tested as a means of preventing breast cancer in women approaching the menopause or who are past the menopause who may be at risk.

As already mentioned, tamoxifen has side-effects in pre-menopausal women. Another drug, gestodene, which has fewer side-effects, is being tested to help prevent breast cancer in pre-menopausal women who may be at risk. It is already used in a low-dose contraceptive pill, but a larger amount of the drug would be needed to prevent breast cancer. The increased dose could also be given in a contraceptive pill, providing cancer protection and birth control for younger women.

Questions Women Most Often Ask About Breast Problems

I'm very worried that my partner will no longer find me attractive now that I've had a mastectomy. What advice can you give me which will help our relationship after surgery?

A loving, supportive relationship will not alter deep down because you have had surgery. But you may have to allow for the anxiety your problem arouses in others close to you; a partner may have difficulty coping with his own feelings as well as yours. Try to communicate how you both feel and offer each other emotional reassurance. The more your partner was involved in your treatment, the more understanding he may be. Some men, however, cannot come to terms with this type of problem, and so you may need support from others.

In some women, the shock and grief at the loss of a breast can be so great that for a time afterwards they can't cope with the thought of having sex. They may not want to be seen naked by their partner or have him caress the other breast. A difficult relationship may crack under such stresses, but a strong one can become stronger.

Sex may restart as part of loving reassurance. As feeling returns during healing, the area will be too tender to bear any pressure, and radiotherapy can increase this sensitivity. This means that lovemaking cannot be so spontaneous, and that positions need to be found which are comfortable for the woman. For instance, if she lies on her side and is entered from behind, this avoids pressure on her chest and arm. It may take time before she can make love in a position where she needs to support herself with her arms; finding suitable positions needs the loving co-operation of her partner. But, as said earlier, a mastectomy is not necessarily a permanent state — breast reconstruction may be possible, and the results can be very good.

Can you describe how breast reconstruction is carried out?

As already mentioned, it may be possible to carry out breast reconstruction at the same time as mastectomy, but often women are advised to have it done about two years later. This allows time to see how the cancer behaves.

If you have had a subcutaneous mastectomy, which leaves the breast skin and nipple intact, a silicone-filled implant can be inserted. The result looks excellent.

Another method is to insert an implant under the pectoralis major chest muscle; the implant is then gradually inflated with silicone or saline solution over a period of weeks. This allows the muscle and skin to stretch, which may cause some discomfort; there is also a risk of infection. In addition, this treatment doesn't always work, because the muscle and skin may be too tight to stretch adequately.

A further type of reconstruction is done by grafting a flap of muscle, fat and skin from elsewhere on the body. It may be taken from the back, abdomen or buttock. The mastectomy incision is opened, the graft fashioned into a breast shape (an implant may be incorporated) and attached on each side to the skin of the chest. A realistic nipple can be made by grafting tissue from the remaining nipple, and the areola created with skin from the thigh or vaginal labia (lips). This results in a breast which looks and feels real, although the nipple will have no sensation. Inevitably, this surgery leaves scars on the breast and at the site from which the graft was removed.

When an implant is used in breast reconstruction, there is the possibility that scar tissue will form round it because the body recognizes it as 'foreign', causing it to harden. Daily massage can help prevent this, or alternatively the implant can be released by 'popping' the scar tissue, which can be done by your doctor while you are under sedation. It's not possible to achieve a perfect match with the other breast, but a reconstructed breast can restore a woman's confidence. It is not the answer for all women, however. Some may have similar feelings about reconstruction as they do about wearing a prosthesis. Or they may not want to go through further complicated surgery which involves another stay in hospital and more discomfort. In some cases it may be the surgeon who is reluctant to carry out a reconstruction, because it can mask a recurrence of cancer in the original site.

How likely is cancer to recur?

A woman who has already had cancer in one breast is at higher risk of developing a malignant tumour in her other breast. This would not be the same cancer recurring, but a new tumour which would be treated in a similar way to the first one. As regards a recurrence or spread of the original cancer, the chances of this diminish with time – the longer you are free of it, the less likely it is to recur. But it is impossible to make anything other than general comments, because cancer may recur even 20 years later.

However, there is now some evidence which shows that the time when surgery was carried out may have some effect on recurrence. It seems that a recurrence is less likely in a pre-menopausal woman if she had surgery in the second half of her menstrual cycle. Hormone levels at this time could have some influence, but other factors may also be involved.

Following the first cancer, you will need regular check-ups, usually at three-month intervals to start with, then every six months, until you may need them only once a year. They will of course remind you of the whole problem, but they are also essential.

Supposing cancer recurs; what can be done then?

A recurrence of cancer is naturally a devastating blow, especially if a woman has already been through surgery, radiotherapy and chemotherapy. But again, these can be powerful weapons in fighting cancer. Even when a complete cure is not possible, the disease can often be effectively controlled for many years.

Would reducing fat in my diet be of significant benefit to me?

The relationship between fat in the diet and breast cancer is still being worked out, but fat is suspect and eating less of it may indeed help lower the risk. Reducing animal fats has definite advantages where heart disease and bowel cancer are concerned. The overall message has to be that a healthier lifestyle can only be of benefit; see Chapter 18.

How can alternative therapies help me cope with breast cancer and the surgery for it?

An alternative practitioner would not try to cure your particular cancer, but would treat the 'whole person'; the aim would be to bring mind and body into better balance by reducing stress and activating your own healing processes. Ways of helping you to become a more fulfilled individual would be explored. 'Alternative' techniques for pain relief and relaxation can help you cope with orthodox treatment; see Chapter 18.

If breast cancer occurs when you are of childbearing age is it safe to have a baby after treatment?

The outcome of breast cancer treatment needs to be assessed. A woman who has had breast cancer must take her surgeon's advice before starting pregnancy.

Is it safe to take the pill or have hormone replacement therapy (HRT) if you have breast problems?

It's thought that the combined oral contraceptive pill can actually provide some protection against benign problems. Where cancer is concerned the picture is less clear, but there is no conclusive evidence that the pill increases the risk.

   HRT* is given to women at the menopause to relieve unpleasant menopausal symptoms*. There is no evidence that it has any influence on benign problems. It would be considered inadvisable for women with a family history of breast cancer to take it, and women who have had breast cancer are usually advised against it. But in all such cases the risks would be carefully weighed against the severity of the menopausal symptoms and the likely benefit to the woman. Where there are no apparent risk factors, careful screening is still carried out before and during HRT.

I have a teenage daughter. What am I to tell her about my cancer? I don't want to frighten her.

All women should be concerned about breast cancer, whether or not they appear to be at risk. Any woman can develop it. Your daughter should know the facts, and how to protect herself through monitoring her own breast health and having medical checks. She should also be encouraged to lead a healthy life, which is the best way we can help ourselves deal with whatever problems come our way.

How can I gain anything from the experience of such a traumatic disease as breast cancer?

Traumatic events often bring about a reassessment of ourselves and our lives, and much can be gained from this. Perhaps the last words of this chapter should go to Diana Moran, the glamorous British TV star who has told her own moving story of her fight against breast cancer.

'The last three months have forced me to stand still. The experience has taught me to be aware of the importance of good health, aware of my own vulnerability and more aware of trivia and insincerity. I've discovered my inner strength and the need to build on it. I've felt the happiness of friendship given and received and the essential inter-dependence of human beings. We all need to communicate, to share our feelings of love, happiness, sadness and compassion, and to spend time listening to others.

'From my brush with cancer, I've learnt to think positively. I've gained confidence, self-respect and inner peace. I feel more strongly than ever before the need to live life for the day, with just a cautious eye to the future. But most of all, I've learnt not take my blessings for granted, and to thank God I'm alive.'

17

RADIOTHERAPY AND
CHEMOTHERAPY

Cancer cells can be destroyed using X-rays* in radiotherapy
and/or drugs in chemotherapy. These treatments may be used
with surgery or on their own if surgery is not feasible.
Radiotherapy and chemotherapy are thought of as being very
unpleasant and producing horrible side-effects, but the treatments themselves are not an ordeal, and there are now much
better ways of dealing with any side-effects that do arise. They
remain powerful weapons against cancer.

The use of radiotherapy and chemotherapy would always be
planned to suit a woman's particular needs, but we can advise on the main approaches, and how best to cope with these
treatments.

*Could you explain more about why radiotherapy and chemotherapy may be
necessary?*

The purpose of cancer surgery is, of course, to remove malignant tissue. Sometimes no further treatment is needed, but
radiotherapy may be used after surgery to destroy any remaining malignant cells. This is because otherwise the cells could
continue to multiply out of control, which is what causes a
tumour (growth or lump) to form in the first place. Prior to
surgery, radiotherapy may be used to shrink a tumour. If
surgery is not possible – perhaps because cancer is advanced, or
the woman is elderly and surgery would be 'too much' for her
– radiotherapy may be carried out on its own. In all cases the

primary tumour site is bombarded with X-rays, and if cancer has spread elsewhere, these other sites may also be treated.

Chemotherapy uses drugs which circulate in the bloodstream and destroy cancer cells that may have spread to other parts of the body. It is used before or after surgery, or if surgery is not possible.

Why don't benign tumours need these treatments?

Benign tumours do not need these treatments because they are 'self-contained': they don't invade surrounding healthy tissue or spread round the body, like cancer. Why cells turn cancerous is not always known, but for further information on the different woman's cancers, see Chapters 12, 13, 14, 15 and 16.

What do these treatments involve?

Your surgeon and a specialist in radiotherapy and chemotherapy would discuss your particular treatment with you beforehand, but here is a general guide to the treatments.

RADIOTHERAPY

Radiotherapy can be carried out internally or externally. The amount of radiation (X-rays) needed must be carefully measured and targeted to minimize damage to surrounding, healthy tissue.

INTERNAL RADIOTHERAPY

This is carried out in hospital. Radioactive implants are placed within the area needing treatment. This may be done before or after surgery on the reproductive organs in the abdomen, or quite often instead of surgery. The implants consist of metal or plastic tubes which contain the radioactive material. They are inserted via the vagina, usually with the patient under general anaesthetic.

The most common reason for this treatment is to combat cervical cancer*. If a woman has not had a hysterectomy* to remove her womb (uterus), a single implant is placed within the cavity of her womb and two additional implants are placed at the top of her vagina against her cervix (the entrance to the womb). If her womb has already been removed, the implants are placed at the top of her vagina; an anaesthetic may not be needed for this insertion.

Once in place, the implants are not painful, although there may be some discomfort. The dosage of radiation required is worked out by a physicist and the radiotherapist who treats you. Treatment may last up to 24 hours.

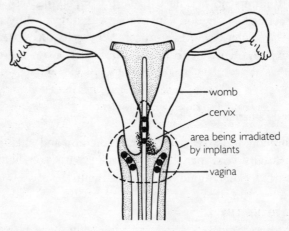

womb
cervix
area being irradiated
by implants
vagina

Radioactive implants are placed against the cervix and inside the womb. This procedure is usually used to treat cervical cancer, either before or instead of surgery.

It is necessary to remain in bed while the implants are inside, to avoid dislodging them accidentally. You would need a catheter (a tube in your urethra) to help you urinate. The main drawback of this treatment is that it can be very boring lying still all the time. Because small amounts of radiation are coming from the implants, you have to be in a specially-protected room on your own during treatment, so that no one else is affected by the radiation. Hospital staff can however come into the room. This is possible because the implants are attached by a slim hose to a sealed lead container, which prevents radiation escaping. The radioactive material, usually in the form of caesium pellets, can be withdrawn from the implants into the container, and reloaded into them again, by remote control (a control button outside the room). You are not radioactive while the pellets are in the container. In some centres the automatic loading device may not be available, in which case the loading will be carried out manually.

When treatment is finished, the implants are carefully pulled out – this may also be uncomfortable if there is an implant in the womb.

How is internal radiotherapy for breast cancer carried out?

Internal radiotherapy for breast cancer is rather different and, at the time of writing, is only available in some hospitals. An implant may be inserted into the breast before surgery, or if surgery is not possible. Insertion is done under general anaesthetic. Most usually, however, the implant is inserted directly after a tumour has been removed by lumpectomy (removal of the tumour only), while the woman is still under anaesthetic.

A breast implant consists of several very thin hollow tubes. These are placed through the tumour 'bed'. They are then filled with radioactive material. When in place, the implant is only a little uncomfortable.

As with internal radiotherapy to the reproductive organs, the woman would be in a specially-protected room on her own for a variable length of time, depending on the radiotherapy needed. But if you are having this treatment, you can move about and leave the room. Again, the implant is attached by a slim hose to a sealed lead container; the radioactive material can be withdrawn and reloaded by remote control. When the radioactive material is in the container, the hose can be detached from the implant, freeing you. But interruptions to treatment should be kept to a minimum. When treatment is over, the tubes are simply pulled out gently, which doesn't hurt. Tiny puncture marks will remain on the skin for a short time, but they soon fade.

The whole course of treatment could be given by this technique while you are in hospital, or part of the treatment may be given using this method, followed by a course of external radiotherapy. Alternatively, the treatment may be in the form of external radiotherapy on its own. Less usually, an implant may be used as a 'booster' after external radiotherapy.

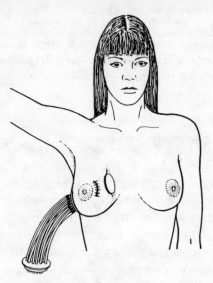

A radioactive implant may be inserted in the breast before surgery or if surgery is not possible. Most usually, though, it is placed through the tumour bed following surgery, as illustrated. Despite appearances, it causes little discomfort.

Would I be in hospital for external radiotherapy?

EXTERNAL RADIOTHERAPY

External radiotherapy to the breast or reproductive organs is usually done on an out-patient basis. You would make visits to the hospital several times a week, spread over several weeks. The area to be treated is marked directly on the skin (and must not be washed off), or on to a plastic wrap which you would wear.

Treatment involves lying on a table under the X-ray machine, which is directed at the area needing radiotherapy. Some women find the equipment frightening, but each session lasts only a few minutes and it's very like having a normal X-ray. You don't see or feel the radiation, nor are you radioactive after treatment sessions. During treatment, you are alone in the room, but the radiographer can observe you through a glass screen or on closed-circuit TV. You can speak to each other via an intercom.

Am I allowed to wash at all during a course of radiotherapy?

Yes, but only splash the area being treated lightly, so as not to remove any markings or cause irritation to your skin by rubbing.

What about chemotherapy; how is this given?

CHEMOTHERAPY

Chemotherapy is usually an out-patient treatment, although overnight stays in hospital may be necessary. It is given as a course of tablets and/or injections: different drugs may be combined in both forms, depending on the woman's needs. Treatment sessions are given over a day or two at a time, and there is a break of about four weeks between each session. The whole course may be spread over several months.

How soon are radiotherapy and chemotherapy started after surgery?

External radiotherapy is started about two or three weeks after surgery, which allows time for healing. Chemotherapy is mapped out according to the schedule for your surgery, and may be started either before or after surgery. If you are having treatment, ensure there will be transport to take you to and from hospital.

Questions Women Most Often Ask About Radiotherapy and Chemotherapy

I'm anxious about the side-effects of these treatments. Why do they occur?

Most side-effects are the result of damage to healthy tissue and, however carefully treatment is given, some damage is unavoidable. Side-effects can occur within a few days, and these depend on how extensive the treatment is. Ask your specialist about the possible side-effects of your particular course of treatment, and what can be done about them.

What side-effects does radiotherapy have?

Following radiotherapy, the most common general side-effect is fatigue. This may not be due entirely to the treatment itself; it could be because you are still recovering from surgery. Ensure that you get plenty of rest.

Radiotherapy to the abdomen can cause nausea, diarrhoea and cystitis (pain and frequency of urination). Certain drugs can counteract these problems. There would not be these side-effects with radiotherapy to the breast.

Vaginal bleeding is quite common following abdominal radiotherapy, so don't be alarmed; it will cease after treatment ends. If the ovaries have not been removed during a hysterecto-my*, radiotherapy will cause them to cease functioning. In a pre-menopausal woman, this can bring on menopausal symptoms*, but in some cases it may be possible to have hormone replacement therapy (HRT)* to relieve them.

The skin over any area being treated by external radiotherapy may redden and blister, although this doesn't always happen. If you have the kind of skin which tolerates the sun well, you're less likely to have a reaction than if you are a pale redhead or blonde. Implants are placed so that any damage to the skin above them is minimal. Applying cortisone ointment or gentian violet can bring relief from a skin reaction, but don't apply cream yourself without medical advice. Radiotherapy to the breast can cause the tissue to thicken and become tender, but this will settle down in time after treatment has finished.

Contrary to popular belief, radiotherapy does not cause hair loss, unless the head is directly treated.

Fortunately, these days most patients receiving radiotherapy do not feel really ill as a result.

Are the side-effects of chemotherapy more severe than those of radiotherapy?

Chemotherapy can have wider-ranging side-effects because the drugs circulate throughout the body. The extent of the side-effects depends on the drugs used. Sometimes they can be more severe than those of radiotherapy, which is why there are breaks in treatment. Nausea and vomiting are quite common, but can be helped by drugs. Tiredness can be the result of anaemia, because anti-cancer drugs reduce the number of blood cells. This also lowers the body's resistance to infection, so you need to live as healthily as possible during treatment; see Chapter 18 for further advice.

Perhaps the most distressing side-effect which often occurs is losing hair from the head, eyebrows and eyelashes. The extent of hair loss also depends on the drugs used. Wearing an 'ice hat' while receiving chemotherapy is a new method which reduces hair loss because it cools the scalp; this contracts the blood vessels and so helps to prevent the drugs from reaching the hair roots. But hair loss is only temporary; it will regrow when treatment is discontinued.

Do I have to have these treatments?

No. As already said in this book, the choice to have any form of treatment is entirely yours. But where radiotherapy and chemotherapy are concerned, you do need to weigh the potential long-term benefits of these treatments against any short-term side-effects. A cure may indeed be possible – cancer is by no means always a 'death sentence'. Even in cases where cancer is advanced, these treatments can often contain the disease and sometimes bring about dramatic improvements.

Can I do anything to help myself cope with cancer treatment?

Yes. A healthy diet will help you combat fatigue. If you have diarrhoea you need to eat 'binding' foods rather than high-fibre ones; see page 269 for dietary advice.

You may also find that alternative therapies, such as relaxation techniques, meditation and acupuncture, are helpful in overcoming nausea and fatigue. There are also ways which may help in resolving negative emotions – despair, grief, anger and anxiety. Alternative therapies can create a sense of inner calm, which can make it much easier to go through radiotherapy and/or chemotherapy.

Using your imagination may enable you to feel positive about cancer treatment and reinforce your desire to be well. The technique known as 'visualization' aims to harness the power of the mind in promoting the benefits of treatment. For instance, this could be done by creating vivid mental images of the radiotherapy and chemotherapy in action destroying your cancer. Read Chapter 18 for more information on alternative therapies.

You are likely to need considerable emotional support if you are being treated for cancer, both to help you cope with treatment and to fight the disease itself. The hospital may organize a support group, or put you in touch with one. There are also well-known cancer charities which offer women counselling and practical help. Those who are caring for you at home may also be in need of support and reassurance; cancer charities can help them, too.

You will, of course, meet other people who are being treated for cancer at your hospital or clinic. It is so often those who, like you, are fighting the disease who have the deepest understanding – and who find strength to help and support not only themselves but others in the same situation.

18

ALTERNATIVE THERAPIES
AND HEALTHIER LIVING

The value of combining orthodox medicine with alternative therapies has become much more widely recognized. The word 'complementary' is now often used instead of 'alternative' because the therapies can 'complement' rather than exclude conventional treatments such as surgery. Where there is co-operation between orthodox and complementary therapies there can also be the best chance of a patient gaining the greatest benefit from both types of medicine. Increasingly, hospitals are opening their doors to alternative/complementary therapists, and doctors becoming more inclined to recommend their treatments. Complementary therapies can enable you to feel altogether better about having surgery, they can help in recovery, and be part of healthier living. Their most important role, however, is in healing by restoring mind, body and spirit to 'wholeness': this is why they are also called 'holistic' or 'whole-person' therapies.

If alternative therapies treat the 'whole person', what effect would this have on my particular problem?

Orthodox medicine concentrates on treating particular health problems by means such as drugs and surgery. Alternative therapies may also improve the specific problem, but most therapies would aim to help you activate your own inner healing power which, it is believed, we all possess.

Could you explain more about how alternative therapies are supposed to work?

The view is that physical disorders can result when mind, body and spirit are 'out of balance'. This may be brought about by a number of factors, such as stress, unhappiness and an unsatisfactory lifestyle. The person is thus in a state of inner disharmony, or 'dis-ease'. Through restoring the balance between mind, body and spirit, alternative therapies work to promote a sense of well-being which can improve every aspect of our lives. Therefore, if you feel calm and optimistic you are more likely to achieve better health than if you are tense and depressed. You are giving your own healing power the chance to work for you.

Medically speaking, this can mean that you are actually strengthening your immune system – the body's natural means of fighting disease and healing itself. This could be why people with a positive attitude often respond so much better to orthodox treatments.

Are alternative therapies a form of self-help?

There is a strong emphasis on self-help, and this can be a great advantage if you're having surgery. It can give you a sense of personal involvement in your own progress. You are not simply in the hands of doctors who can apply high-tech treatments aimed at 'making you well'. You are actively participating in the process by doing something for yourself.

I am facing surgery. How can alternative therapies help me to help myself?

Before surgery, they can be used to relieve stress and anxiety, enabling you to face it feeling more relaxed and positive. You are likely to experience less pain in this state. And a therapy such as acupuncture can have a direct pain-relieving effect. Following surgery, they can help to promote vitality and speed recovery.

Which alternative therapies should I try, and how do I find a therapist?

There is a wide range of alternative therapies, and it's a matter of deciding which therapy, or combination of therapies, will benefit you most. An alternative therapist may practise several types of therapy. Your doctor may be able to recommend suitable therapies, as already mentioned, and put you in touch with a therapist. If you are having hospital treatment, find out whether the hospital provides any complementary therapies, or has contact with outside therapists. Some doctors, nurses and other health care professionals have also trained in alternative/complementary medicine, and so can help you themselves.

If you are seeking help, contact the organizations which represent the types of therapy you wish to try (see the Useful Addresses section). They will put you in touch with the nearest fully trained and reputable therapist who, as a member of an organization, will be bound by its code of practice. Alternative therapists should not advise you against having orthodox treatment, nor can they offer a cure. However, they are generally as committed to helping their patients as is any doctor. It is also just as vital to have a good personal rapport with a therapist as it is to be on good terms with your doctor.

Can you describe the therapies which could be most useful to me as a surgical patient?

In the space of a chapter it's only possible to give an introduction to the therapies which could be most useful to you, and which are likely to be easily available. The books listed in the References and Further Reading section will give you more detailed information.

YOGA

Yoga is probably the best known and most widely available alternative therapy, although it could be more accurately described as an ancient Indian philosophy. Harmony between mind, body and spirit is central to Yoga (Yoga is Sanskrit for 'union'). An important part of the Yoga philosophy is a system of exercises which provide considerable therapeutic benefits. This system consists of pranayama (breathing exercises), asanas (postures), and meditation.

Yoga is usually taught in classes; there is likely to be one in your area. You can of course also learn it from books and tapes, but a good teacher is invaluable. Once you have learned the basics, you can practise on your own. Yoga can help you prepare for surgery, and it can also be used in hospital and during recovery.

If you feel tense and afraid, the breathing exercises can reduce your natural stress reaction by slowing your heart rate and lowering blood-pressure. This has a calming effect. There is a way of breathing which can be carried out anywhere, as follows.

Keeping your back straight, breathe in deeply, filling the lungs, using your diaphragm (the muscle which lies between your chest and abdominal cavity). Go on breathing deeply, slowly and regularly; this is how you should always breathe. It prevents the shallow, rapid 'upper chest' breathing (hyperventilation) which results from stress and is so bad for the heart and other organs.

The postures are designed to improve your suppleness and muscular control. Together with correct breathing, they are a preparation for meditation.

The purpose of meditation is to relax the mind and create inner peace, not to dwell on problems and anxieties. There are several ways of meditating, which are touched on later in this chapter. It can certainly help you in hospital, and also to cope with treatments such as radiotherapy* and chemotherapy*.

THE ALEXANDER TECHNIQUE
This is becoming increasingly popular, and is often described as being the Western version of Yoga. It is taught on a one-to-one basis; it should not be difficult to find a teacher locally. The Technique is based on the view that virtually all of us have learned to use our bodies incorrectly. Physical and emotional ills can result from bad posture and awkward movements – and the misuse of our bodies can also be an expression of mental stresses which in themselves produce serious ill health.

It is a gentle therapy which brings the whole body into proper alignment and teaches correct breathing. Your teacher would help you by literally moving your body into the right positions.

The mind is approached through re-educating the body as a means of achieving physical and mental well-being. The release of tension and sense of balance the Technique promotes can help you prepare for surgery and recover afterwards.

ACUPUNCTURE

Acupuncture is another well-known alternative therapy which is now much more widely accepted. Valuable in relieving stress and pain, its benefits to a surgical patient are obvious. It came to the West from China, where it has many uses, including that of an anaesthetic; major operations are carried out with the patients fully conscious and completely pain-free. It isn't used in surgery here, but is gaining ground in hospitals as a means of post-operative pain relief; it can also quell nausea following an anaesthetic.

The side-effects of radiotherapy and chemotherapy – such as nausea and fatigue – can also be alleviated by acupuncture. In China it has been found that when acupuncture is combined with radiotherapy and chemotherapy to treat advanced cancer, survival rates seem to improve.

In the West, modern, medically trained acupuncturists, who may work in hospitals, adhere to the basics of acupuncture: the insertion of very fine sterile needles into specific points on the body. You might feel a little pain on insertion, or just a pin-prick, although some people experience only numbness and others feel no sensation at all. A mild electric current may be applied to the needles to cause them to vibrate, which makes the treatment more effective. All the patient feels is the vibra-tion. The needles can remain in place from a few minutes to about half an hour.

According to ancient tradition, the needle points occur on lines called meridians, along which flows the universal energy known as Chi. The twin forces of Yang and Yin are an impor-tant part of this concept. They complement each other, creating a balance in all living things. For instance, Yang represents such universal forces as the sun, warmth and movement; Yin stands for its opposite, i.e. the moon, coolness, repose and moisture. Yang is often referred to as being 'masculine' and Yin 'feminine'. It is when the energy flow – the Yang and Yin – becomes unbalanced within us that ill health and pain may ensue. Acupuncture frees the energy flow along the meridians and restores our natural balance.

The modern scientific view is that the meridians coincide with the main nerve pathways, and that 'needling' them intercepts pain messages to the brain, so that no pain is felt. Acupuncture may also work to release the body's natural painkilling hormones, called endorphins.

If you visit a traditional holistic acupuncturist before surgery or during convalescence, you would be treated in a more elaborate way than if you received the therapy in more orthodox surroundings such as in hospital. This traditional method could involve the use of herbs. Your diet, lifestyle and emotional attitudes would be discussed, to see if they could be improved.

SHIATSU AND ACUPRESSURE
These are forms of acupuncture, carried out without needles. Finger pressure is used on the meridians to bring relief, and you can learn to treat yourself. As with acupuncture, it results in feelings of relaxation and comfort.

REFLEXOLOGY
Reflexology involves foot massage. Different areas of the feet are thought to relate to various parts of the body. Massage is believed to free energy channels throughout the body, with benefits similar to those of acupuncture and acupressure.

HOMOEOPATHY
Homoeopathy is an alternative therapy which has acquired respectability, particularly in Britain, where it has Royal patronage. Homoeopathic doctors may also be qualified in orthodox medicine.

Homoeopathic medicine treats 'like with like'. In other words, symptoms are seen as the body's attempts to heal itself, and not as a sign of ill health. A homoeopathic doctor will therefore work 'with' symptoms, unlike an orthodox doctor, who will use medicine and treatments to dispel them. Another basic principle of homoeopathy is that 'less is more': the more a remedy is diluted – and the less there apparently is of it – the more potent it becomes. Remedies are often derived from plants, and are taken by mouth. Some therapists combine homoeopathy with acupuncture (this is known as homoeopuncture), the needles being first dipped in homoeopathic remedies before insertion.

Practically all diseases and disorders can be treated by homoeopathy. In deciding on a treatment to suit you, a homoeopathic doctor would be as interested in your personality as your health problem. Although the remedies are very different to orthodox ones, they are aimed at stimulating the immune system, and so can be used alongside orthodox medical treatments. Homoeopathy is a complex kind of medicine which is not easily explained. It is also regarded with much scepticism in certain quarters, but none the less its supporters find it very helpful.

AROMATHERAPY

Aromatherapy is massage using essential oils extracted from plants. It is a very beneficial kind of massage for those with health problems. A trained aromatherapist can apply oils such as rose, lavender, bergamot and geranium, which are believed to help relieve anxiety and depression. Essential oils can also be used in the bath to relieve fatigue and loss of appetite following surgery; these may include rosemary, melissa and sandalwood. However, you would need to consult your doctor before receiving any massage treatment if you are having cancer surgery, radiotherapy and/or chemotherapy.

Some hospital nurses are trained in aromatherapy, and find that patients who receive this type of massage sleep better and experience less pain than those who do not.

HYPNOTHERAPY

Hypnotherapy relaxes the mind, reduces tension, and relieves pain. A trance-like state is induced, which is like being between sleeping and waking. What usually happens is that the hypnotherapist sits opposite or near you and talks to you in soft, slow, persuasive tones. While this happens, you may be asked to focus your eyes on a particular object. Once you are under hypnosis the therapist can 'suggest' to you that you are relaxing and that any pain or discomfort you are feeling is lessening. The effects of his or her suggestions can carry over into consciousness for a time. Hypnotherapy worries some people, because they feel that under hypnosis the mind is 'open' to the influence of the hypnotherapist, who might abuse this power. It would hardly be sensible, however, for a reputable hypnotherapist to do this.

Interestingly, this power of suggestion is also used in orthodox medicine. At Glasgow Royal Infirmary in Scotland, 'positive suggestion' tapes are played to patients while they are under general anaesthetic. Hysterectomy patients receive messages such as 'Your operation will be successful, you feel warm and comfortable, any pain will not concern you.' Women who have been played these messages have needed less post-operative pain relief than those who have not been played any.

VISUALIZATION

This can enable you to activate your own healing powers by using your imagination. Cancer patients in particular can benefit from it. How it is used depends on the woman's personal interests and her attitude to the disease. For instance, a woman who enjoys gardening could imagine (or visualize) her surgery, radiotherapy and/or chemotherapy as being like a powerful garden tool which destroys cancer cells – the invading weeds – and leaves her body a well-tended flower bed.

Some women, however, do not think of their cancer as an invading enemy. They may see it as a part of themselves which needs sorting out. They might then visualize their body as a house needing a thorough clean and tidy, or an office with a chaotic computer system. Treatment could be seen as giving them the means of restoring order. Visualization is actually a form of meditation.

MEDITATION

Meditation can be approached in many ways. It can be done in a group with a teacher, or on your own. We have mentioned

Yoga meditiation, which aims to relax the mind and create inner peace. Simply concentrating on breathing slowly, deeply and steadily is a start, or the mind can be focused on a colour or sound. Hindu meditation, for example, concentrates the mind on 'mantras', or sacred words.

COUÉISM

Meditation may lie between hypnosis and visualization, as it does in Couéism. This is named after the nineteenth-century French apothecary, Emile Coué, who devised that most famous of all Western mantras, 'Every day, in every way, I am getting better and better.' Its purpose is not to make you consciously 'will' yourself better; the mantra, repeated often enough, is meant to permeate the deeper levels of your unconscious and stimulate your imagination, so that you 'see' yourself getting better. Contemplating Coué's words can be done anytime, anywhere, and could help you during post-operative treatment and in recovery.

AUTOGENIC TRAINING

This is related to both Couéism and hypnosis. It is a further way of achieving complete relaxation through activating your imagination. This can be brought about by concentrating on messages such as 'My arms are heavy and warm, my legs are heavy and relaxed, my heartbeat is slow and regular,' and ending with 'I am at peace.' Your whole body can be relaxed in this way. If you're facing tests or procedures which are to be carried out under local anaesthetic, or without anaesthetic, it could be an excellent way to deal with 'pre-op nerves'. There are books and tapes based on this method which can be helpful, but it is always better to learn autogenics from personal instruction in a class.

PRAYER

Prayer is a profound form of meditation when it is no longer done on an overtly conscious level. Not everyone will feel comfortable with the idea of meditation. For them, simply praying (alone or with someone else) before an operation may be comforting, even to those without formal beliefs. And knowing that others are praying for you, or wishing you well in their thoughts, is what 'absent healing' is all about.

MEDITATION-IN-MOTION

Meditation-in-motion reaches the mind and spirit through the body. You have probably seen Chinese people on film performing graceful movements in an idyllic landscape. This is T'ai Chi. The movements create balance and tranquillity, the physical peace leading to a spiritual calm. Through the movements you become 'tuned-in' to Chi, the universal energy which flows through all living things. This builds energy within you, so that the graceful movements become effortless. T'ai Chi can be performed with a partner by alternately 'pushing hands' and yielding in flowing motion. It is now taught quite widely in adult education colleges, and would help you regain strength and confidence when recovering from surgery.

DANCE THERAPY

Dance therapy is as much about self-expression as balance. It needs to be performed in a group, and is now offered in some hospitals and clinics. The purpose is to 'loosen up' your body as a way of freeing your mind and allowing the expression of emotion through movement. Often the dancers form a circle; they may hold hands and make other supportive gestures to one another. The dance may be done to music or to the dancers' own rhythms.

This therapy allows 'dance dramas', which permit people to express their fears, anger or sorrow. Patients often feel they can relate the onset of their health problems to a traumatic experience, a personal loss, or a period of stress and frustration. It is possible that such experiences may influence hormonal balance. The hypothalamus is an area of the brain which registers our emotions and co-ordinates our hormonal and nervous systems. Women's health problems are often related to hormonal imbalance*. Although a direct connection between physical illness and negative emotions cannot be proved, it cannot be ruled out, either.

Dance therapy can be a way of coming to terms with, and exorcising, damaging experiences and feelings. It is gaining orthodox approval for precisely these reasons: patients who are allowed this emotional release in a supportive group are more likely to respond well to more orthodox medical treatments.

HEALING

Healing, and the many ways it can be administered, is a vast subject. Again, we can only touch on some of the approaches here. Probably best known is spiritual or faith healing. This implies a belief in God: the healer is the means of conveying the divine healing love. It used to be thought that only 'special' people had healing powers. Now there is also the view that not only do we all possess the ability to heal ourselves, we can also heal others, and that no traditional religious belief is necessary. Love is central. Unconditional love activates our healing energies and channels them towards others.

How is healing carried out? Healers will have their own individual approaches, but generally healing involves the 'laying-on' of hands. You may sit or lie down, and the healer may start by placing his or her hands on your head, or holding them above it. The hands are then moved down your body – more often they are held over it rather than placed directly on it. They may be passed over your whole body, or held above specific 'trouble spots'. Therapeutic Touch and the Japanese Reiki are forms of healing through touch. There is no doubt that healing can produce powerful responses. People may literally 'feel the energy' from the healer's hands, as a tingling sensation or a glowing warmth – or even very powerfully, like an electric shock (but without any harmful effects).

Does it work? Healers will emphasize that healing is not about producing 'miracle cures', although sometimes remarkable improvements occur. Healing is intended to awaken a person's desire to heal him- or herself. Ill health may sometimes be like a slow form of suicide. A person is healed, without necessarily being cured, if depression or despair can be replaced by peace and hope.

Healers are allowed to visit patients and to practise in some hospitals. Their help could be of benefit throughout surgical treatment of all kinds.

COUNSELLING

This is now so universally available that it scarcely counts as an 'alternative therapy' any more, although it is the basis of many such therapies. It can be carried out on a one-to-one basis, or in a support group where the group members are actually counselling each other. The aim is to help you deal with the personal problems connected with ill health and its treatment. Those who have had counselling do tend to feel that it has been worthwhile, and there is evidence that they benefit more from medical treatment as a result.

Counselling is often directed at helping you to lead a more fulfilling life. As has been stated repeatedly, stress and negative emotions may make us more liable to ill health because they depress our immune system or – in alternative terms – impair our energy flow. There is also the view that it is not stress itself, but a person's reaction to it, which lowers resistance to ill health. It is considered more a matter of 'personality type'.

This view is thought by some experts to be particularly relevant to cancer patients. The 'cancer-prone personality' belongs to a woman who bottles up her emotions, lacks creative outlets, and may be over-anxious to please others. Counsellors who hold this view would try to help such a woman find ways of expressing herself and realizing her creative potential. The causes of illness may be complex, however, and perhaps related to some aspects of life which are beyond our immediate control, such as heredity and environment. Whatever the causes might be, patients should not feel guilty or inadequate for being ill.

What about the practical side of 'healthier living', such as diet. As a surgical patient, would I benefit from an 'alternative' diet?

NATUROPATHY

Naturopathy is an alternative approach very much concerned with diet as a part of overall healthier living, the emphasis being on fresh food and fresh air. Health farms offer naturopathic therapy. You could go to one when recovering from surgery, if your doctor considers it a good idea and you can afford it.

Naturopathic diets vary, but they are often vegetarian, and much of the food is eaten raw. Alcohol and smoking are usually banned or at least strongly discouraged.

Such a diet can be difficult to keep up when you are at home with people whose tastes may be very different, however, and it is not suitable for every patient. Some general advice which is easy to follow may therefore be helpful. Here is a guide to the balance of foods you need daily to build vitality before and after surgery, and to maintain your health.

- Vegetables, salads, and fruit: 55 per cent
- Lean meat, fish, low-fat dairy produce, beans, peas, lentils, and nuts: 20 per cent
- Cereals, brown rice, wholemeal bread, and pasta: 20 per cent
- Non-animal fats (spreads, cooking oil): 5 per cent

Avoid sugary, starchy foods, which increase your weight and have little nutritional value.

This balance contains the right proportion of vitamins and minerals, as well as fibre to aid digestion and prevent constipation. It is also low in fat. If you are having radiotherapy* and/or chemotherapy*, which can cause diarrhoea, you need less fibre and more 'binding' foods, such as eggs, cheese, fish, and lean meat.

If your appetite suffers following surgery, the best thing to do is eat small amounts often. Alcohol need not be avoided; a little can stimulate the appetite. A glass of sherry before your main meal is a well-known appetizer, and may even be available in hospital if you ask for it. Smoking, however, depresses the immune system, and is a total enemy of health.

Do I need extra vitamins? Should I take vitamin supplements?

It depends on what your doctor advises. Taken in the recommended dosage, a course of vitamin pills can help 'build you up' after surgery if you don't feel much like eating. But all vitamins are found in fresh foods, and this is the best way to obtain them. Avoid overcooking fresh foods, as this reduces their nutritional value.

There is some evidence that extra vitamin C can help in healing and may also benefit cancer patients. It's found mainly in citrus fruits and green leafy vegetables. Vitamin A (found in carrots, broccoli and liver) is also thought beneficial for cancer patients. Too much vitamin A can be harmful, however, because unlike vitamin C, any surplus is not excreted by the body. Vitamin B6 (found in wholemeal bread, rice, liver and fish) is thought to benefit women with benign breast problems and to help strengthen the immune system.

How much exercise do I need?

This book gives advice on specific exercises which will help in recovery where appropriate. How much general exercise you should take depends on your overall state of health. People with health problems may benefit most from exercise that does not overstress the body, such as swimming, walking and gentle stretching exercises, which can be done every day.

Will the 'healing' effects of alternative therapies make me a fitter person?

Alternative therapies aim to do much more than simply restore physical fitness, but Yoga, the Alexander Technique, T'ai Chi and dance therapy will benefit you on this level without overstressing your body.

Whether you are facing surgery or recovering from it, our hope is that this book will help you to be healed on all levels.

REFERENCES AND FURTHER READING

Health Guides

Bradford, Nikki, *The Well Woman's Self Help Directory*, Sidgwick & Jackson, 1990.
British Medical Association, *The British Medical Association Complete Family Health Encyclopedia*, Dorling Kindersley, 1990.
Llewellyn-Jones, Derek, *The A-Z of Women's Health*, Oxford University Press, 1990.
——, *Everywoman – A Gynaecological Guide for Life*, Faber & Faber, 1989.
Phillips, Angela, and Rakusen, Jill, *The New Our Bodies, Ourselves*, Penguin, 1989.
Stanway, Dr Andrew, *A Dictionary of Operations*, Paladin, 1981.

Period Problems

Graham, Judy, *Evening Primrose Oil*, Thorsons, 1989.
Kingston, Beryl, *Lifting the Curse*, Sheldon Press, 1984.
Melville, Arabella, *Natural Hormone Health*, Thorsons, 1990.

Infertility

Anderson, Mary, *Infertility – A Guide for the Anxious Couple*, Faber & Faber, 1987.
Barker, Dr Graham H., *Overcoming Infertility*, Hamlyn, 1990.
Gunn, Dr Alexander, *Infertility – A Practical Guide to Coping*, The

Crowood Press, 1988.
Hawkridge, Caroline, Understanding Endometriosis, Macdonald
Optima, 1989.
Neuberg, Roger, Infertility, Thorsons, 1991.
Winston, Robert, Getting Pregnant, Anaya, 1989.
——, Infertility – A Sympathetic Approach, Macdonald Optima, 1987.

Pregnancy and Childbirth

Anderson, Mary, Pregnancy After Thirty, Faber & Faber, 1984.
Bostock, Yvonne, and Jones, Maggie, Now or Never? Having a Baby
Later in Life, Thorsons, 1987.
Duffett-Smith, Tricia, You and Your Caesarean Birth, Sheldon Press,
1985.
Reader, F., and Savage, W., Coping with Caesarean and Other Difficult
Births, Macdonald, 1983.

Termination/Abortion

Frater, Alison, and Wright, Catherine, Coping with Abortion,
Chambers, 1986.
Kenyon, Edwin, The Dilemma of Abortion, Faber & Faber, 1986.
Neustatter, Angela, and Newson, Gina, Mixed Feelings – The
Experience of Abortion, Pluto Press, 1986.
Pipes, Mary, Understanding Abortion, The Women's Press, 1986.
Winn, Denise, Experiences of Abortion, Macdonald Optima, 1988.

Miscarriage

Jones, Wendy, Miscarriage – Overcoming the Physical and Emotional
Trauma, Thorsons, 1990.
Kohner, Nancy, and Henley, Alix, When a Baby Dies – The Experience
of Late Miscarriage, Stillbirth and Neonatal Death, Thorsons, 1991.
Leroy, Margaret, Miscarriage, Macdonald Optima, 1988.
Oakley, Ann, McPherson, Ann, and Roberts, Helen, Miscarriage,
Penguin, 1990.

Sterilization

Dolto, Dr C., Schiffmann, Dr A., and Bello, P., *How to Get Pregnant and How Not to*, Sheldon Press, 1985.

Goldstein, Marc, and Feldberg, Michael, *The Vasectomy Book – A Complete Guide to Decision-making*, Turnstone Press, 1985.

Hayman, Suzie, *Vasectomy and Sterilization – What You Need to Know*, Thorsons, 1989.

Women's Cancers

Clyne, Rachel, *Cancer – Your Life, Your Choice*, Thorsons, 1989.

Dawson, Donna, *Women's Cancers*, Piatkus, 1990.

Faulder, Carolyn, *The Women's Cancer Book*, Virago, 1989.

LeShan, Lawrence, *Cancer as a Turning Point*, Gateway Books, 1990.

Shaw, Clare, and Hunter, Maureen, *The Cancer Special Diet Cookbook*, Thorsons, 1991.

Sikora, Professor Karol, and Thomas, Dr Hilary, *Fight Cancer*, BBC Books, 1989.

Stroud, Marion, *Face to Face with Cancer*, Lion Publishing, 1988.

CERVICAL CANCER AND PRE-CANCER

Chomet, Dr Jane, and Chomet, Julian, *Cervical Cancer*, Thorsons, 1989.

Quilliam, Susan, *Positive Smear*, Penguin, 1989.

Singer, Albert, and Szarewski, Dr Anne, *Cervical Smear Test*, Macdonald Optima, 1988.

BREAST CANCER AND BENIGN PROBLEMS

Baum, Professor Michael, *Breast Cancer – the Facts*, Oxford University Press, 1988.

Cirket, Cath, *A Woman's Guide to Breast Health*, Thorsons, 1989.

Cochrane, John, and Szarewski, Dr Anne, *The Breast Book*, Macdonald Optima, 1989.

Gilbert, Dr Patricia, *What Every Woman Should Know About Her Breasts*, Sheldon Press, 1986.

Moran, Diana, *A More Difficult Exercise*, Bloomsbury, 1989.

Wallis, Claudia, and Nash, J. Madeleine, 'A Puzzling Plague', *Time*, January 14, 1991.

Hysterectomy

Dickson, Anne, and Henriques, Nikki, Hysterectomy – the Positive Recovery Plan, Thorsons, 1989.
Hayman, Suzie, Hysterectomy – What it is, and How to Cope with it Successfully, Sheldon Press, 1986.
Hufnagel, Dr Vicki, No More Hysterectomies, Thorsons, 1990.
Webb, Ann, Experiences of Hysterectomy, Macdonald Optima, 1989.
Winn, Denise, 'Pain: Who Needs It?' The Sunday Times colour supplement, 24th February 1991.

The Menopause

Gorman, Teresa (MP), and Whitehead, Dr Malcolm, The Amarant Book of Hormone Replacement Therapy, Pan Books, 1989.
Henriques, Nikki, and Dickson, Anne, Menopause – The Woman's View, Thorsons, 1987.
Ojeda, Linda, Menopause Without Medicine, Thorsons, 1990.
Shreeve, Dr Caroline M., Overcoming the Menopause Naturally, Arrow Books, 1987.

Alternative Therapies

Bartlett, E.G., Healing Without Harm, Paperfronts, Elliot Right Way Books, 1985.
Drake, Jonathan, Body Know-how – A Practical Guide to the Use of the Alexander Technique in Everyday Life, Thorsons, 1991.
Feldenkrais, Moshe, Awareness Through Movement, Thorsons, 1991.
Gaier, Harald, Thorsons Encyclopedic Dictionary of Homoeopathy, Thorsons, 1991.
Goldsmith, Joel K., The Art of Meditation, Thorsons, 1991.
Grist, Liz, A Woman's Guide to Alternative Medicine, Fontana, 1986.
Hodgkinson, Liz, The Alexander Technique, Piatkus, 1988.
Humphrey, Naomi, Meditation – The Inner Way, Thorsons, 1987.
Kenyon, Dr Julian, Acupressure Techniques, Thorsons, 1987.
Lewith, George T., Acupuncture, Thorsons, 1982.
Macrae, Janet, Therapeutic Touch, Penguin, 1987.

Marcus, Dr Paul, *Thorsons Introductory Guide to Acupuncture*, Thorsons, 1991.

Martin, Simon, 'Shiatsu – Healing at a Touch', *Here's Health*, December 1990.

Newman Turner, Roger, *Naturopathic Medicine*, Thorsons, 1990.

O'Brien, Paddy, *A Gentler Strength – the Yoga Book for Women*, Thorsons, 1991.

Ousby, William J., *The Theory and Practice of Hypnotism*, Thorsons, 1990.

Page, Michael, *Visualization – The Key to Fulfilment*, Thorsons, 1990.

Tisserand, Maggie, *Aromatherapy for Women*, Thorsons, 1990.

Healthier Living

Kirsta, Alix, *The Book of Stress Survival*, Unwin Hyman, 1986.

Mayes, Adrienne, *The A-Z of Nutritional Health*, Thorsons, 1991.

Newhouse, Sonia, *The Complete Natural Food Reckoner*, Thorsons, 1991.

Ridgway, Judy, *The Vitamin and Mineral Special Diet Cookbook*, Thorsons, 1990.

Westcott, Patsy, *Alternative Healthcare for Women*, Thorsons, 1991.

Sex Manuals

Anand, Margo, *The Art of Sexual Ecstasy*, Thorsons, 1990.

Brown, Paul, and Faulder, Carolyn, *Treat Yourself to Sex*, Penguin, 1989.

Cauthery, Dr Philip, and Stanway, Drs Andrew and Penny, *The Complete Book of Love and Sex*, Century, 1986.

Kitzinger, Sheila, *Woman's Experience of Sex*, Penguin, 1985.

Yaffé, Maurice, Fenwick, Elizabeth, and Rosen, Raymond C., *Sexual Happiness – A Practical Approach*, Dorling Kindersley, 1986.

USEFUL ADDRESSES

If you wish to contact a support group, counselling service or an alternative/complementary therapist, your doctor, local hospital, 'well woman' or family planning clinic can often provide you with the information and advice you need. If necessary, you can also contact the following organizations, bearing in mind that this list cannot be comprehensive.

Australia

ALTERNATIVE THERAPIES
Australian Natural Therapists Ass.
PO Box 522
Sutherland
New South Wales 2232
Tel: (02) 521 2063
Provides information, advice and referrals throughout Australia.

Australian Traditional Medicine
  Society
Suite 3, 1st Floor
120 Blaxland Road
Ryde
New South Wales 2112
Tel: (02) 808 2825
Provides information and publishes a directory of organizations and practitioners.

Blackmore's Naturopathic Clinic &
  Research Centre
Suite 17
47 Neridan Street
Chatswood
New South Wales 2067
Tel: (02) 411 1099
Offers counselling and treatment.

Complementary & Environmental
  Medicine Centre
41 Boundary Street
Rushcutters Bay
Sydney
New South Wales 2001
Tel: (02) 380 5233/5474
Staffed by both complementary therapists and doctors, the centre offers counselling and treatment.

CANCER CARE
Australian Cancer Society
Angus and Coote Building
500 George Street
Sydney
and
GPO Box 4708
Sydney
New South Wales 2001
Tel: (02) 267 1944

Information and advice on all aspects
of cancer. List of inter-state member
organizations. Publishes national journal: *Cancer Forum*.

INFORMATION AND COUNSELLING
Inter-state women's health centres
providing information and counselling on all aspects of women's
health concerns

Adelaide   Women's   Community
    Health Centre
64 Pennington Terrace
North Adelaide
South Australia 5006
Tel (toll free): (008) 182 098

Leichhardt Women's Health Centre
55 Thornley Street
Leichhardt
New South Wales 2040
Tel: (02) 560 3011

Women's Health Care House
92 Thomas Street
W. Perth
Western Australia 6005
Tel: (09) 321 2383

Women's Health Centre
PO Box 237
North Hobart
Tasmania 7002
Tel: (002) 28 0997

Women's Health Information Centre
Royal Women's Hospital
132 Grattan Street
Carlton
Victoria 3053
Tel: (03) 344 2007/2199

Women's Health Information Service
Healthsharing Women
318 Little Bourke Street
Melbourne
Victoria 3000
Tel: (03) 663 4457
Women's health centre with national
links.

Women's Health Information
    Resource Collective
653 Nicholson Street
Carlton North
Victoria 3054
Tel: (03) 387 8702
Booklets and tapes available on all
aspects of women's health concerns.

Women's Health Service
GPO Box 825
Canberra
Australian Capital Territory 2601
Tel: (062) 45 4411

Women's Information Centre
Casuarina Plaza
Casuarina
Northern Territory 0810
Tel: (089) 27 7166

Women's Information Service
280 Adelaide Street
Brisbane
Queensland 4000
Tel: (07) 229 1264

Britain

ALTERNATIVE THERAPIES

The Institute for Complementary
  Medicine
4 Tavern Quay
Sweden Gate
Surrey Quays
London SE16 1QZ
Tel 071–237 5165
Library, information service, referrals.
Publishes *The Journal of Complementary Medicine*.

COUNSELLING

Women's Health
52–54 Featherstone Street
London EC1Y 8RT
Tel: 071–251 6580
Provides advice and information; puts
women in touch with health care
organizations throughout the country; publishes a newsletter.

Canada

ALTERNATIVE THERAPIES

Acupuncture Foundation of Canada
2 Sheppard Avenue East
1004 North York
Ontario
M2N 5Y7

Association of Naturopathic
Practitioners
921–17 Avenue South West
Calgany
Alberta
T2T 0A4

COUNSELLING

Canadian PID Society
PO Box 33804
Station D
Vancouver, B.C.
V6J 4L6
Tel: (604) 684–5704
Advice and support for PID (pelvic
inflammatory disease) sufferers.

Pacific Post Partum Society
Suite 104–1416 Commercial Drive
Vancouver, B.C.
V5L 3X9
Tel: (604) 255–7999
Advice and support following child-
birth.

Vancouver Women's Health
Collective
Suite 302
1720 Grant Street
Vancouver, B.C.
V5L 2Y7
Tel: (604) 255–8285
Health information centre, publica-
tions list, counselling, medical refer-
ral, educational workshops.

Women's Health Clinic
3rd Floor
419 Graham Avenue
Winnipeg, Manitoba
R3C 0M3
Tel: (204) 947–1517
Health information centre, counselling, support groups, publications
list, educational workshops, medical
treatment.

New Zealand

ALTERNATIVE THERAPIES
Auckland College of Classical
Homoeopathy
PO Box 19–502
Avondale
Auckland 7
Tel: 8289 700
Counselling and treatment of
women's health problems, especially
infertility.

New Zealand Natural Health
Practitioners Accreditation Board
PO Box 37–491
Auckland
Publishes a nationwide register of
natural therapists who have met the
Board's standards.

South Pacific College of Natural
Therapeutics (NZ) Inc
PO Box 11311
Ellerslie
Auckland
Tel: (09) 579 4997
Gives advice and puts women in
touch with an appropriate organiza-
tion and practitioner.

INFORMATION
Federation of Women's Health
Councils
PO Box 853
Auckland
Puts women in touch with health
care services throughout the country.
Write for information.

South Africa

Medical Association of South Africa
PO Box 20272
Alkantrant
Pretoria 0005
Tel: (12) 47–6101
Information on women's health care
resources throughout the country.

United States

ALTERNATIVE THERAPIES
Touch for Health Foundation
1174 North Lake Avenue
Pasadena, CA 91104
Tel: (818) 794–1181
International educational foundation
dedicated to research and teaching in
touch-healing.

CANCER CARE
American Cancer Society (ACS)
1599 Clifton Road, N.E.
Atlanta, GA 30329
Tel (national toll-free number): 1-
800-227-2345
Access to a comprehensive cancer
information database. Information
also available by post.

Natonal Cancer Care Foundation and
National Alliance of Breast Cancer
Organizations
1180 Avenue of the Americas
New York, NY 10036
Tel: (212) 221–3300

Dedicated to addressing the emotional, social and financial problems
brought about by cancer. Provides
information and education on cancer.

Y – ME National Organization for
Breast Cancer
Information & Support
18220 Harwood Avenue
Homewood, IL 60430
Tel (national toll-free hotlines): 800-
221-2141 (9–5 weekdays); 708-799-
8228 (24 hours)
Provides information, counselling,
medical referral and emotional support to women concerned about or
diagnosed with breast cancer.
Education workshops and newsletter.

COUNSELLING
Center for Medical Consumers
237 Thompson Street
New York, NY 10012
Tel: (212) 674-7105
General advice and information on
women's health concerns.

Endometriosis Association
PO Box 92187
Millwaukee, WI 53202
Tel: (414) 355 2200
Advice and support for emdometrio-
sis sufferers.

Santa Cruz Women's Health Center
250 Locust Street
Santa Cruz, CA 95060
Tel: (408) 427 – -3500
General advice and information ser-
vice.

FERTILITY ADVICE
Resolve
5 Water Street
Arlington, Mass 02174
Tel: (617) 643–2424
Advice and information on infertility.

INDEX